MW00875107

Long COVID Supplements

© Copyright: Steven Magee 2023

Edition 1

Cover Picture: SARS-CoV-2 as seen by a cryo-electron tomography scan by Nanographics.

https://nanographics.at/projects/coronavirus-3d/

Contents

Introduction

I developed a flu-like sickness that was followed by years of long COVID symptoms. My mental and physical health seriously degraded after the flu-like sickness and I was largely a medical mystery to the doctors that were treating me. The prescription medications and medical devices would make me sicker, not better.

Using nutritional supplements and lifestyle changes I started to see beneficial health improvements and my health recovered sufficiently to resume a normal life again. I am sharing the fruits of my discoveries with you, so you can work with your doctor on improving your own health. I got smart and my smart techniques are in this book!

At the time of writing, the COVID-19 pandemic was in its fourth year and long COVID was prevalent in the population. The nutritional supplements discussed in this book are being linked to improved health outcomes in both conditions.

Scientific research papers that discuss the nutritional supplements I used to improve my long COVID symptoms are presented. My supplementation protocols for my long COVID symptoms were developed from supplementation experimentation and medical research that was freely available on the internet. Altitude tests to cause hypoxia throughout the body were performed on the island of Hawaii from 2021 to 2023 to confirm the supplements prevented hypoxic sickness from the lower atmospheric oxygen levels.

The three supplement protocols detailed in this book were developed during the COVID-19 pandemic. The long COVID symptoms I was displaying significantly subsided by using the three supplement protocols. I have much better mental and physical health today. I look better too!

This book contains the very latest research on health and the human environment. It should be viewed as the current ideas and the contents are subject to review by the medical community. The author and publisher accept no liability whatsoever for any of the contents and the book is published in the spirit of unrestricted access to the latest ideas and medical theories in a changing world. These are experimental health techniques and the long term side effects are unknown.

You should always consult with a licensed and certified medical professional on any aspects of health, sickness or disease.

"During my time of need, the medical system failed me."

Steven Magee

Long COVID

Long COVID or Post-COVID Conditions...Some people who have been infected with the virus that causes COVID-19 can experience long-term effects from their infection, known as Long COVID or Post-COVID Conditions (PCC). Long COVID is broadly defined as signs, symptoms, and conditions that continue or develop after initial COVID-19 infection. This definition of Long COVID was developed by the Department of Health and Human Services (HHS) in collaboration with CDC and other partners. People call Long COVID by many names, including Post-COVID Conditions, long-haul COVID, post-acute COVID-19, long-term effects of COVID, and chronic COVID. The term post-acute sequelae of SARS CoV-2 infection (PASC) is also used to refer to a subset of Long COVID...People with Long COVID can have a wide range of symptoms that can last weeks, months, or even years after infection. Sometimes the symptoms can even go away and come back again. For some people, Long COVID can last weeks, months, or years after COVID-19 illness and can sometimes result in disability...

- General symptoms (Not a Comprehensive List):
    - Tiredness or fatigue that interferes with daily life.
    - Symptoms that get worse after physical or mental effort (also known as "post-exertional malaise").
    - Fever.
- Respiratory and heart symptoms:
    - Difficulty breathing or shortness of breath.
    - Cough.
    - Chest pain.
    - Fast-beating or pounding heart (also known as heart palpitations).
- Neurological symptoms:

- ○ Difficulty thinking or concentrating (sometimes referred to as "brain fog").
- ○ Headache.
- ○ Sleep problems.
- ○ Dizziness when you stand up (lightheadedness).
- ○ Pins-and-needles feelings.
- ○ Change in smell or taste.
- ○ Depression or anxiety.
- Digestive symptoms:
  - ○ Diarrhea.
  - ○ Stomach pain.
- Other symptoms:
  - ○ Joint or muscle pain.
  - ○ Rash.
  - ○ Changes in menstrual cycles.

...People with Long COVID may develop or continue to have symptoms that are hard to explain and manage. Clinical evaluations and results of routine blood tests, chest X-rays, and electrocardiograms may be normal. The symptoms are similar to those reported by people with myalgic encephalomyelitis/chronic fatigue syndrome (ME/CFS) and other poorly understood chronic illnesses that may occur after other infections. People with these unexplained symptoms may be misunderstood by their healthcare providers, which can result in a long time for them to get a diagnosis and receive appropriate care or treatment...Some people, especially those who had severe COVID-19, experience multiorgan effects or autoimmune conditions with symptoms lasting weeks, months, or even years after COVID-19 illness. Multi-organ effects can involve many body systems, including the heart, lung, kidney, skin, and brain. As a result of these effects, people who have had COVID-19 may be more likely to develop new health conditions such as diabetes, heart conditions, blood clots, or neurological conditions compared with people who have not had COVID-19. https://www.cdc.gov/coronavirus/2019-ncov/long-term-effects/index.html

Long COVID: An overview...Fatigue, cough, chest tightness, breathlessness, palpitations, myalgia and difficulty to focus are symptoms reported in long COVID. It could be related to organ damage, post viral syndrome, post-critical care syndrome and others. Clinical evaluation should focus on identifying the pathophysiology, followed by appropriate remedial measures. In people with symptoms suggestive of long COVID but without known history of previous SARS-CoV-2 infection, serology may help confirm the diagnosis.

https://pubmed.ncbi.nlm.nih.gov/33892403/

Pathophysiology and mechanism of long COVID: a comprehensive review...After almost 2 years of fighting against SARS-CoV-2 pandemic, the number of patients enduring persistent symptoms long after acute infection is a matter of concern...Apart from long-term organ damage, many hints suggest that specific mechanisms following acute illness could be involved in long COVID symptoms...Long-COVID is a multisystem disease that develops regardless of the initial disease severity. Its clinical spectrum comprises a wide range of symptoms. The mechanisms underlying its pathophysiology are still unclear. Although organ damage from the acute infection phase likely accounts for symptoms, specific long-lasting inflammatory mechanisms have been proposed, as well.

https://pubmed.ncbi.nlm.nih.gov/35594336/

Long COVID: major findings, mechanisms and recommendations...Long COVID is an often debilitating illness that occurs in at least 10% of severe acute respiratory syndrome coronavirus 2 (SARS-CoV-2) infections. More than 200 symptoms have been identified with impacts on multiple organ systems. At least 65 million individuals worldwide are estimated to have long COVID, with cases increasing daily. Biomedical research has made substantial progress in identifying various pathophysiological changes and risk factors and in characterizing the illness; further, similarities with other viral-onset illnesses such as myalgic encephalomyelitis/chronic fatigue syndrome and postural orthostatic tachycardia syndrome have laid the groundwork for research in the field. In this review, we explore the current literature and highlight key findings, the overlap with other conditions, the variable onset of symptoms, long COVID in children and the impact of vaccinations.

https://pubmed.ncbi.nlm.nih.gov/36639608/

Symptoms and risk factors for long COVID in non-hospitalized adults...Outcomes included 115 individual symptoms, as well as long COVID, defined as a composite outcome of 33 symptoms by the World Health Organization clinical case definition. Cox proportional hazards models were used to estimate adjusted hazard ratios (aHRs) for the outcomes. A total of 62 symptoms were significantly associated with SARS-CoV-2 infection after 12 weeks. The largest aHRs were for anosmia (aHR 6.49, 95% CI 5.02-8.39), hair loss (3.99, 3.63-4.39), sneezing (2.77, 1.40-5.50), ejaculation difficulty (2.63, 1.61-4.28) and reduced libido (2.36, 1.61-3.47). Among the cohort of patients infected with SARS-CoV-2, risk factors for long COVID included female sex, belonging to an ethnic minority, socioeconomic deprivation, smoking, obesity and a wide range of comorbidities. The risk of developing long COVID was also found to be increased along a gradient of decreasing age. SARS-CoV-2 infection is associated with a plethora of symptoms that are associated with a range of sociodemographic and clinical risk factors.

https://pubmed.ncbi.nlm.nih.gov/35879616/

Post-COVID-19 Syndrome...Since the beginning of the coronavirus disease 2019 (COVID-19) pandemic, many individuals have reported persistent symptoms and/or complications lasting beyond 4 weeks, which is now called post-COVID-19 syndrome. SARS-CoV-2 is a respiratory coronavirus that causes COVID-19, and injury to the lungs is expected; however, there is often damage to numerous other cells and organs, leading to an array of symptoms. These long-term symptoms occur in patients with mild to severe COVID-19; currently, there is limited literature on the potential pathophysiological mechanisms of this syndrome... Although studies examining the pathophysiology of post-COVID-19 syndrome are still relatively few, there is growing evidence that this is a complex and multifactorial syndrome involving virus-specific pathophysiological variations that affect many mechanisms but specifically oxidative stress, immune function, and inflammation. Further research is needed to elucidate the pathophysiology, pathogenesis, and longer term consequences involved in post-COVID-19 syndrome.

https://pubmed.ncbi.nlm.nih.gov/34653099/

Long COVID, a comprehensive systematic scoping review... The predominant symptoms were: fatigue, breathlessness, arthralgia, sleep difficulties, and chest pain. Recent reports also point to the risk of long-term sequela with cutaneous, respiratory, cardiovascular, musculoskeletal, mental health, neurologic, and renal involvement in those who survive the acute phase of the illness.

https://pubmed.ncbi.nlm.nih.gov/34319569/

Epidemiology, Symptomatology, and Risk Factors for Long COVID Symptoms: Population-Based, Multicenter Study... Background: Long COVID induces a substantial global burden of disease. The pathogenesis, complications, and epidemiological and clinical characteristics of patients with COVID-19 in the acute phase have been evaluated, while few studies have characterized the epidemiology, symptomatology, and risk factors of long COVID symptoms. Its characteristics among patients with COVID-19 in the general population remain unaddressed. Objective: We examined the prevalence of long COVID symptoms, its symptom patterns, and its risk factors in 4 major Chinese cities in order to fill the knowledge gap. Methods: We performed a population-based, multicenter survey using a representative sampling strategy via the Qualtrics platform in Beijing, Shanghai, Guangzhou, and Hong Kong in June 2022. We included 2712 community-dwelling patients with COVID-19 and measured the prevalence of long COVID symptoms defined by the World Health Organization (WHO), and their risk factors. The primary outcomes were the symptoms of long COVID, with various levels of impact. A descriptive analysis of the prevalence and distribution of long COVID symptoms according to disease severity was conducted. A sensitivity analysis of increasing the number of long COVID symptoms was also conducted. Univariate and multivariate regression analyses were performed to examine the risk factors of severe long COVID symptoms, including age, gender, marital status, current occupation, educational level, living status, smoking habits, monthly household income, self-perceived health status, the presence of chronic diseases, the use of chronic medication, COVID-19 vaccination status, and the severity of COVID-19. Results: The response rate was 63.6% (n=2712). The prevalence of long COVID, moderate or severe long COVID, and severe long COVID was 90.4% (n=2452), 62.4% (n=1692), and 31.0% (n=841), respectively. Fatigue (n=914, 33.7%), cough (n=865, 31.9%), sore throat (n=841, 31.0%), difficulty in concentrating (n=828, 30.5%), feeling of anxiety (n=817, 30.2%), myalgia (n=811, 29.9%), and arthralgia (n=811, 29.9%) were the most common severe long COVID symptoms. From multivariate regression analysis, female gender (adjusted odds ratio [aOR]=1.49, 95% CI 1.13-1.95); engagement in transportation, logistics, or the discipline workforce (aOR=2.52, 95% CI 1.58-4.03); living with domestic workers (aOR=2.37, 95% CI 1.39-4.03); smoking (aOR=1.55, 95% CI 1.17-2.05); poor or very poor self-perceived health status (aOR=15.4, 95% CI 7.88-30.00); ≥3 chronic diseases (aOR=2.71, 95% CI 1.54-4.79); chronic medication use (aOR=4.38, 95% CI 1.66-11.53); and critical severity of COVID-19 (aOR=1.52, 95% CI 1.07-2.15) were associated with severe long COVID. Prior vaccination with ≥2 doses of COVID-19 vaccines was a protective factor (aOR=0.35-0.22, 95% CI 0.08-0.90). Conclusions: We examined the prevalence of long COVID symptoms in 4 Chinese cities according to the severity of COVID-19. We also evaluated the pattern of long COVID symptoms and their risk factors. These findings may inform early identification of patients with COVID-19 at risk of long COVID and planning of rehabilitative services.

https://pubmed.ncbi.nlm.nih.gov/36645453/

Long-COVID and Post-COVID Health Complications: An Up-to-Date Review on Clinical Conditions and Their Possible Molecular Mechanisms...The COVID-19 pandemic has infected millions worldwide, leaving a global burden for long-term care of COVID-19 survivors. It is thus imperative to study post-COVID (i.e., short-term) and long-COVID (i.e., long-term) effects, specifically as local and systemic pathophysiological outcomes of other coronavirus-related diseases (such as Middle East Respiratory Syndrome (MERS) and Severe Acute Respiratory Syndrome (SARS)) were well-cataloged. We conducted a comprehensive review of adverse post-COVID health outcomes and potential long-COVID effects. We observed that such adverse outcomes were not localized. Rather, they affected different human systems, including: (i) immune system (e.g., Guillain–Barré syndrome, rheumatoid arthritis, pediatric inflammatory multisystem syndromes such as Kawasaki disease), (ii) hematological system (vascular hemostasis, blood coagulation), (iii) pulmonary system (respiratory failure, pulmonary thromboembolism, pulmonary embolism, pneumonia, pulmonary vascular damage, pulmonary fibrosis), (iv) cardiovascular system (myocardial hypertrophy, coronary artery atherosclerosis, focal myocardial fibrosis, acute myocardial infarction, cardiac hypertrophy), (v) gastrointestinal, hepatic, and renal systems (diarrhea, nausea/vomiting, abdominal pain, anorexia, acid reflux, gastrointestinal hemorrhage, lack of appetite/constipation), (vi) skeletomuscular system (immune-mediated skin diseases, psoriasis, lupus), (vii) nervous system (loss of taste/smell/hearing, headaches, spasms, convulsions, confusion, visual impairment, nerve pain, dizziness, impaired consciousness, nausea/vomiting, hemiplegia, ataxia, stroke, cerebral hemorrhage), (viii) mental health (stress, depression and anxiety). We additionally hypothesized mechanisms of action by investigating possible molecular mechanisms associated with these disease outcomes/symptoms. Overall, the COVID-19 pathology is still characterized by cytokine storm that results to endothelial inflammation, microvascular thrombosis, and multiple organ failures.

https://www.ncbi.nlm.nih.gov/pmc/articles/PMC8072585/

Long COVID: pathophysiological factors and abnormalities of coagulation...Acute COVID-19 infection is followed by prolonged symptoms in approximately one in ten cases: known as Long COVID. The disease affects ~65 million individuals worldwide. Many pathophysiological processes appear to underlie Long COVID, including viral factors (persistence, reactivation, and bacteriophagic action of SARS CoV-2); host factors (chronic inflammation, metabolic and endocrine dysregulation, immune dysregulation, and autoimmunity); and downstream impacts (tissue damage from the initial infection, tissue hypoxia, host dysbiosis, and autonomic nervous system dysfunction). These mechanisms culminate in the long-term persistence of the disorder characterized by a thrombotic endothelialitis, endothelial inflammation, hyperactivated platelets, and fibrinaloid microclots. These abnormalities of blood vessels and coagulation affect every organ system and represent a unifying pathway for the various symptoms of Long COVID.

https://www.ncbi.nlm.nih.gov/pmc/articles/PMC10113134/

Prevalence and characteristics of long COVID in elderly patients: An observational cohort study of over 2 million adults in the US...Incidence of long COVID in the elderly is difficult to estimate and can be underreported. While long COVID is sometimes considered a novel disease, many viral or bacterial infections have been known to cause prolonged illnesses. We postulate that some influenza patients might develop residual symptoms that would satisfy the diagnostic criteria for long COVID, a condition we call "long Flu."...We observed that about 30% of hospitalized COVID-19 patients developed long COVID. In a similar proportion of patients, long COVID-like symptoms (long Flu) can be observed after influenza, but there are notable differences in symptomatology between long COVID and long Flu. The impact of long COVID on healthcare utilization is higher than long Flu.

https://pubmed.ncbi.nlm.nih.gov/37068113/

Long-COVID Symptoms in Individuals Infected with Different SARS-CoV-2 Variants of Concern: A Systematic Review of the Literature...This systematic review compares the prevalence of long-COVID symptoms according to relevant SARS-CoV-2 variants in COVID-19 survivors...The sample included 355 patients infected with the historical variant, 512 infected with the Alpha variant, 41,563 infected with the Delta variant, and 57,616 infected with the Omicron variant...The prevalence of long-COVID was higher in individuals infected with the historical variant (50%) compared to those infected with the Alpha, Delta or Omicron variants. It seems that the prevalence of long-COVID in individuals infected with the Omicron variant is the smallest, but current data are heterogeneous, and long-term data have, at this stage, an obviously shorter follow-up compared with the earlier variants. Fatigue is the most prevalent long-COVID symptom in all SARS-CoV-2 variants, but pain is likewise prevalent. The available data suggest that the infection with the Omicron variant results in fewer long-COVID symptoms compared to previous variants...It appears that individuals infected with the historical variant are more likely to develop long-COVID symptomatology.

https://pubmed.ncbi.nlm.nih.gov/36560633/

COVID-19 and its long-term sequelae: what do we know in 2023?...Post-viral syndrome is a well-known medical condition characterized by different levels of physical, cognitive, and emotional impairment that may persist with fluctuating severity after recovering from an acute viral infection. Unsurprisingly, COVID-19 may also be accompanied by medium- and long-term clinical sequelae after recovering from a SARS-CoV-2 infection. Although many clinical definitions have been provided, "long-COVID" can be defined as a condition occurring in patients with a history of SARS-CoV-2 infection, developing 3 months from the symptoms onset, persisting for at least 2 months, and not explained by alternative diagnoses. According to recent global analyses, the cumulative prevalence of long-COVID seems to range between 9% and 63%, and is up to 6-fold higher than that of similar postviral infection conditions. Long-COVID primarily encompasses the presence of at least 1 symptom, such as fatigue, dyspnea, cognitive impairment / brain fog, postexertional malaise, memory issues, musculoskeletal pain / spasms, cough, sleep disturbances, tachycardia / palpitations, altered smell / taste perception, headache, chest pain, and depression. The most important demographic and clinical predictors to date are female sex, older age, cigarette smoking, pre-existing medical conditions, lack of COVID-19 vaccination, infection with pre-Omicron SARS-CoV-2 variants, number of acute phase symptoms, viral load, severe / critical COVID-19 illness, as well as invasive mechanical ventilation. Concerning the care for long-COVID patients, the greatest challenge is the fact that this syndrome cannot be considered a single clinical entity, and thus it needs an integrated multidisciplinary management, specifically tailored to the type and severity of symptoms.

https://pubmed.ncbi.nlm.nih.gov/36626183/

Long Covid: Untangling the Complex Syndrome and the Search for Therapeutics...Long Covid can affect anyone who has previously had acute COVID-19. The root causes of this syndrome are still unknown, and no effective therapeutics are available. This complex syndrome, with a wide array of symptoms, is still evolving. Given the dire situation, it is important to identify the causes of Long Covid and the changes occurring within the immune system of affected patients to figure out how to treat it. The immune system intersects with the persistent viral fragments and blood clots that are implicated in this syndrome; understanding how these complex systems interact may help in untangling the puzzling physiopathology of Long Covid and identifying mitigation measures to provide patients some relief. In this paper, we discuss evidence-based findings and formulate hypotheses on the mechanisms underlying Long Covid's physiopathology and propose potential therapeutic options.

https://pubmed.ncbi.nlm.nih.gov/36680082/

"Long COVID is not new, as it was previously reported as 'Post-Viral Illness' which is also called 'Long Flu'."

Steven Magee

Nutrition

Nutritional deficiencies that may predispose to long COVID...Multiple nutritional deficiencies (MND) confound studies designed to assess the role of a single nutrient in contributing to the initiation and progression of disease states. Despite the perception of many healthcare practitioners, up to 25% of Americans are deficient in five-or-more essential nutrients. Stress associated with the COVID-19 pandemic further increases the prevalence of deficiency states. Viral infections compete for crucial nutrients with immune cells. Viral replication and proliferation of immunocompetent cells critical to the host response require these essential nutrients, including zinc. Clinical studies have linked levels of more than 22 different dietary components to the likelihood of COVID-19 infection and the severity of the disease. People at higher risk of infection due to MND are also more likely to have long-term sequelae, known as Long COVID.

https://pubmed.ncbi.nlm.nih.gov/36920723/

Long-Term Evolution of Malnutrition and Loss of Muscle Strength after COVID-19: A Major and Neglected Component of Long COVID-19...Results: Of 549 consecutive patients hospitalized for COVID-19 between 1 March and 29 April 2020, 23.7% died and 288 patients were at home at D30 post-discharge. At this date, 136 of them (47.2%) presented persistent malnutrition, a significant decrease in muscle strength or a PS $\geq$ 2. These patients received dietary counseling, nutritional supplementation, adapted physical activity guidance or physiotherapy assistance, or were admitted to post-care facilities. At 6 months post-discharge, 91.0% of the 136 patients (n = 119) were evaluated and 36.0% had persistent malnutrition, 14.3% complained of a significant decrease in muscle strength and 14.9% had a performance status > 2. Obesity was more frequent in patients with impairment than in those without (52.8% vs. 31.0%;

$p = 0.0071$), with these patients being admitted more frequently to ICUs (50.9% vs. 31.3%; $p = 0.010$). Among those with persistent symptoms, 10% had psychiatric co-morbidities (mood disorders, anxiety, or post-traumatic stress syndrome), 7.6% had prolonged pneumological symptoms and 4.2% had neurological symptoms. Conclusions: Obese subjects as well as patients who have stayed in intensive care have a higher risk of functional loss or undernutrition 6 months after a severe COVID infection. Malnutrition and loss of muscle strength should be considered in the clinical assessment of these patients.

https://pubmed.ncbi.nlm.nih.gov/34836219/

The Role of Nutrients in Prevention, Treatment and Post-Coronavirus Disease-2019 (COVID-19)...the safe intake of micro- and/or macro-nutrients can be useful either for preventing infection and supporting the immune response during COVID-19, as well as in the post-acute phase, i.e., "long COVID", that is sometimes characterized by the onset of various long lasting and disabling symptoms. The aim of this review is to focus on the role of nutrient intake during all the different phases of the disease, including prevention, the acute phase, and finally long COVID... In this review we have discussed a number of studies showing that nutrition may play an important role in influencing both the susceptibility and the clinical course of COVID-19 and long COVID, as is already known for other viral diseases. We have shown that nutritional status plays a pivotal role in the function of the immune system, supporting both innate and adaptive immunity, influencing the proliferation and activity of immune cells. Furthermore, we highlighted that nutrients play a role in reducing inflammation. They inhibit leukocyte chemotaxis, inflammatory cytokine production, and T lymphocyte reactivity. Moreover, they give rise to resolvins and protectins, which participate in the resolution of inflammation by normalizing excessive immune reactions. In addition, they are essential for keeping intact and functioning tissue barriers. Finally, some of them seem to influence viral replication and they have even been shown to have a neuroprotective effect in long COVID, by decreasing cognitive decline.

https://www.ncbi.nlm.nih.gov/pmc/articles/PMC8912782/

Dietary Recommendations for Post-COVID-19 Syndrome...At the beginning of the coronavirus disease (COVID-19) pandemic, global efforts focused on containing the spread of the virus and avoiding contagion. Currently, it is evident that health professionals should deal with the overall health status of COVID-19 survivors. Indeed, novel findings have identified post-COVID-19 syndrome, which is characterized by malnutrition, loss of fat-free mass, and low-grade inflammation. In addition, the recovery might be complicated by persistent functional impairment (i.e., fatigue and muscle weakness, dysphagia, appetite loss, and taste/smell alterations) as well as psychological distress. Therefore, the appropriate evaluation of nutritional status (assessment of dietary intake, anthropometrics, and body composition) is one of the pillars in the management of these patients. On the other hand, personalized dietary recommendations represent the best strategy to ensure recovery. Therefore, this review aimed to collect available evidence on the role of nutrients and their supplementation in post-COVID-19 syndrome to provide a practical guideline to nutritionists to tailor dietary interventions for patients recovering from COVID-19 infections.

https://pubmed.ncbi.nlm.nih.gov/35334962/

Acute malnutrition recovery rates improve with COVID-19 adapted nutrition treatment protocols in South Sudan: a mixed methods study...Within the context of the ongoing COVID-19 pandemic in South Sudan, improved recovery, default, and non-responder rates were observed following adoption of changes to nutrition protocols. Policymakers in South Sudan and other resource-constrained settings should consider if simplified nutrition treatment protocols adopted during COVID-19 improved performance and should be maintained in lieu of reverting to standard treatment protocols.

https://pubmed.ncbi.nlm.nih.gov/36906599/

"Long term malnutrition can be the outcome of a viral infection."

Steven Magee

Supplements

Nutritional Support During Long COVID: A Systematic Scoping Review...Nutritional rehabilitation was an important aspect of recovery from severe inflammation, malnutrition, and sarcopenia in hospital rehabilitation programs. Current gaps in the literature include a potential role for anti-inflammatory nutrients such as the omega 3 fatty acids, which are currently undergoing clinical trials, glutathione-boosting treatments such as N-acetylcysteine, alpha-lipoic acid, or liposomal glutathione in long COVID, and a possible adjunctive role for anti-inflammatory dietary interventions. This review provides preliminary evidence that nutritional interventions may be an important part of a rehabilitation program for people with severe long COVID symptomatology, including severe inflammation, malnutrition, and sarcopenia.

https://pubmed.ncbi.nlm.nih.gov/37102680/

Long COVID and its Management...It is recommended to obtain a complete assessment including full blood count, renal function test, C-reactive protein, liver function test, thyroid function, hemoglobin A1c (HbA1c), vitamin D, magnesium, B12, folate and ferritin levels...In long COVID, chronic inflammation provokes multi-organ damage and exacerbates pre-existing conditions. Dietary supplements, such as vitamins and minerals, contain anti-inflammatory and anti-oxidative components, so they have become potential treatments for long COVID. A pilot study demonstrates that multivitamin supplements improve clinical symptoms among long COVID patients. In addition, a commercial plant extract supplement from Panax ginseng and Eleutherococcus senticosus effectively relieved post-COVID fatigue and improved health status in 201 long COVID patients. Nicotinamide ribose, a form of vitamin B3, is being examined for its effects of ameliorating cognitive dysfunctions and chronic fatigue in two clinical trials (NCT04809974, NCT04604704). Essential fatty acids, such as omega-3 (Eicosatetraenoic acid - EPA + docosahexaenoic acid - DHA), are also being examined for their functions in long COVID symptoms (NCT05121766). Long COVID patients often have dysregulated lipid oxidation and lactate accumulation during physically active state, indicating compromised mitochondrial function. The mitochondrial dysfunction in long COVID shares similar symptoms as the ones observed in Myalgic encephalomyelitis/chronic fatigue syndrome (ME/CFS). Supplementation with Coenzyme Q10 (CoQ10) is found to reduce fatigue frequency and relieve oxidative stress among ME/CFS patients. Currently, high-dose CoQ10 treatment is being investigated in a Phase II clinical trial in long COVID patients (NCT04960215). Dietary supplements may also have beneficial effect in modulating systemic inflammation and immunity. Natural flavonoids such as luteolin and quercetin are promising immunomodulatory agents which have showed inhibitory effects on mast cells. The influence of microbiota on immunity is well known, and long COVID leads to significant changes in gut flora. Dietary pro-biotics and pre-biotics are being evaluated on their impacts on clinical symptoms, immune function and biomarkers in long COVID patients (NCT04813718).

https://www.ncbi.nlm.nih.gov/pmc/articles/PMC9305273/

Fatigue in Covid-19 survivors: The potential impact of a nutritional supplement on muscle strength and function...Fatigue with reduced tolerance to exercise is a common persistent long-lasting feature amongst COVID-19 survivors...After 28 days of nutritional supplementation with Apportal® in COVID-19 survivors affected by fatigue with reduced tolerance to exercise, we found a significant improvement in means of muscle strength and physical performance, associated with enhancement of self-rated health status.

https://pubmed.ncbi.nlm.nih.gov/36184207/

Note: The vitamins and minerals contained in ApportAL® are useful to perform four important macro-functions:

- Immune: Vitamin C, Vitamin D, Zinc Sucrosomial®, Iron Sucrosomial® and Selenium Sucrosomial® promote normal immune system function.

- Antioxidant: the presence of Selenium Sucrosomial®, Vitamin E, Vitamin C, Zinc Sucrosomial®, Tocotrienols, Coenzyme Q10 and Lycopene helps protect cells from oxidative stress.

- Energising: Vitamin B1, Vitamin C, Magnesium Sucrosomial®, Iodine Sucrosomial®, Iron Sucrosomial® and Vitamin PP contribute to normal energy metabolism and the reduction of tiredness and fatigue, while Taurine and Ginseng help to increase energy and vitality.

- Muscular: Magnesium Sucrosomial® and Vitamin D contribute to the maintenance of normal muscle function. Carnitine and Arginine are also added to these micronutrients.

https://www.pharmanutra.it/en/brand/pharmanutra/italiano-apportal/

"Prolonged sickness often results from nutritional deficiencies and can be offset through supplementing the diet."

Steven Magee

Multivitamins

Examining the role of micronutrients on improving long COVID sleep-related symptoms...There is evidence to suggest that sleep-related symptoms associated with long COVID, such as fatigue and poor sleep quality, are associated with inflammation. Zinc, vitamins C, D and polyphenols all have the potential to improve both inflammation and sleep quality to alleviate symptoms. Future research should further examine these micronutrients in the context of long COVID to improve sleep and quality of life.

https://pubmed.ncbi.nlm.nih.gov/36539931/

COVID-19: Role of Nutrition and Supplementation...current research indicates that supplementation with multiple micronutrients could be considered important both in the prevention and in the management of the COVID-19 infection. Particular attention should be paid to the substances that play an important role in the regulation of the immune response, considering the possibility of reducing the risk of infection, and, at the same time, improving the health status of COVID-19 patients. The micronutrients with the strongest evidence for immune support are vitamins C, D, and zinc. To date, evidence has been published about the pivotal role of vitamin D: Its deficiency has been associated with increased susceptibility to respiratory infections. Considering that the main pathway of the SARS-CoV-2 infection is at the lung level, it is reasonable that the use of vitamin D supplements could improve the health status of COVID-19 patients, reducing the risk of infection for healthy individuals, helping COVID-19 survivors in the recovery of their lifestyle...the role of probiotics should be better studied in order to reduce the adverse effects at gastrointestinal levels of the COVID-19 infection...it is well described that the worst outcomes occur in subjects with one or more comorbidities. Furthermore, each comorbidity is strictly related to metabolic diseases: For example, the overweight or obese subject has a high risk of developing the severe form of SARS-CoV-2 infection. For these reasons, it is important to take into account the influence of lifestyle habits, such as unhealthy diets, on COVID-19 susceptibility and recovery. In addition, the large number of subjects who recover from COVID-19 could lead to a spike in chronic medical diseases. These conditions could be further exacerbated by a poor diet regimen. Therefore, in consideration of the data discussed in this review, it should be recommended that subjects should avoid eating foods containing high amounts of saturated fat and sugar; contrariwise, it is desirable that they consume high amounts of fiber, whole grains, unsaturated fats, and antioxidants to enhance immune function.

https://www.ncbi.nlm.nih.gov/pmc/articles/PMC8002713/

Proposal of a food supplement for the management of post-COVID syndrome...A vast majority of COVID-19 patients experience fatigue, extreme tiredness and symptoms that persist beyond the active phase of the disease. This condition is called post-COVID syndrome. The mechanisms by which the virus causes prolonged illness are still unclear. The aim of this review is to gather information regarding post-COVID syndrome so as to highlight its etiological basis and the nutritional regimes and supplements that can mitigate, alleviate or relieve the associated chronic fatigue, gastrointestinal disorders and continuing inflammatory reactions. Naturally-occurring food supplements, such as acetyl L-carnitine, hydroxytyrosol and vitamins B, C and D hold significant promise in the management of post-COVID syndrome. In this pilot observational study, we evaluated the effect of a food supplement containing hydroxytyrosol, acetyl L-carnitine and vitamins B, C and D in improving perceived fatigue in patients who recovered from COVID-19 but had post-COVID syndrome characterized by chronic fatigue. The results suggest that the food supplement could proceed to clinical trials of its efficacy in aiding the recovery of patients with long COVID.

https://pubmed.ncbi.nlm.nih.gov/34890036/

"Multivitamins can help offset nutritional deficiencies."

Steven Magee

B Vitamins

A Google search of "long covid pubmed 2023 B complex" produced no relevant findings. It appears there is little research being done in this area.

"Vitamin B complex can be better than a multivitamin."

Steven Magee

Vitamin B6

Potential Role of Vitamin B6 in Ameliorating the Severity of COVID-19 and Its Complications...Vitamin B6 is a water-soluble vitamin found in various foods such as fish, whole grains, and banana. There are six isoforms of B6 vitamers. Among these, pyridoxal 5'-phosphate is the most active form that acts as a coenzyme in various enzymatic reactions. There is growing evidence that vitamin B6 exerts a protective effect against chronic diseases such as cardiovascular diseases (CVD) and diabetes by suppressing inflammation, inflammasomes, oxidative stress, and carbonyl stress. Additionally, vitamin B6 deficiency is associated with lower immune function and higher susceptibility to viral infection. In view of these information, we postulated potential role of vitamin B6 in ameliorating the severity of COVID-19 and its complications...Accumulating evidence suggests that vitamin B6 supplementation may be useful for COVID-19 patients with low vitamin B6 status.

https://www.ncbi.nlm.nih.gov/pmc/articles/PMC7658555/

"Vitamin B6 has a protective effect on the body."

Steven Magee

Biotin (B7)

Importance of Dietary Changes During the Coronavirus Pandemic: How to Upgrade Your Immune Response...both nutritional excess and deficiency are associated with immunodeficiency, adequate nutrition leading to an optimally functioning immune system may be associated with better outcomes with regards to preventing infection and complications of COVID-19, as well as developing a better immune response to other pathogenic viruses and microorganisms...Vitamin B7 has a crucial role in nutrition and an important effect in immunometabolism. In fact, by being an essential cofactor for acetyl-CoA carboxylase and fatty acid synthase, this vitamin is used by the body to metabolize carbohydrates, fats, and amino acids (229). The AI of vitamin B7 is 12–30 μg/day for adults (150). Vitamin B7 deficiency induces Th1- and Th17-mediated pro-inflammatory responses in human CD4+ T lymphocytes (230). In the same context, a diet rich in vitamin B7 has anti-inflammatory effects and inhibits the activation of the transcription of NF-ϰB and thus inhibits the secretion of pro-inflammatory cytokines such as TNF-α, IL-1, IL-6, and IL-8.

https://www.ncbi.nlm.nih.gov/pmc/articles/PMC7481450/

The snapshot of metabolic health in evaluating micronutrient status, the risk of infection and clinical outcome of COVID-19...Metabolic disruption, proceeding from modifiable factors, has been proposed as a significant risk factor accounting for infection susceptibility, disease severity and risk for post-COVID complications...adequate energy production for immune cell activities, gut microbiota composition, fatty acid oxidation, reactive oxygen species (ROS) generation, T cell differentiation and regulation of inflammatory signaling, all comprise key components of B-vitamin mediated monitoring. The sufficiency of beneficial gut microflora can be indirectly evaluated through the levels of vitamin B7 (biotin). This vitamin is endogenously produced by probiotic gastrointestinal bacteria and is required as a coenzyme to promote fatty acid biosynthesis, gluconeogenesis and amino acid metabolism. Biotin-dependent 3-methylcrotonyl-CoA carboxylase promotes leucine catabolism, and decreased enzymatic capacity is associated with the accumulation of 3-methyl crotonic acid and 3-hydroxyisovaleric acid in the biological fluids.

https://www.ncbi.nlm.nih.gov/pmc/articles/PMC8234252/

"Vitamin B7 assists in the metabolization of carbohydrates, fats, and amino acids in the body."

Steven Magee

Folate (B9)

A Google search of "long covid pubmed 2023 B-9 B9 Folate" produced no relevant findings. It appears there is little research being done in this area.

"Approximately 4% of hospitalized COVID-19 patients have folate deficiency."

Steven Magee

Vitamin B12

COVID-19: A methyl-group assault?...The socio-economic implications of COVID-19 are devastating. Considerable morbidity is attributed to 'long-COVID' – an increasingly recognized complication of infection. Its diverse symptoms are reminiscent of vitamin B12 deficiency, a condition in which methylation status is compromised. We suggest why SARS-CoV-2 infection likely leads to increased methyl-group requirements and other disturbances of one-carbon metabolism. We propose these might explain the varied symptoms of long-COVID. Our suggested mechanism might also apply to similar conditions such as myalgic encephalomyelitis/chronic fatigue syndrome. The hypothesis is evaluable by detailed determination of vitamin B12 and folate status, including serum formate as well as homocysteine and methylmalonic acid, and correlation with viral and host RNA methylation and symptomatology. If confirmed, methyl-group support should prove beneficial in such individuals...We suggest that SARS-CoV-2 induces an increased demand for methyl-groups whilst simultaneously impairing their supply due to viral-induced oxidative stress. The biochemical implications of our hypothesis might explain the diverse symptoms experienced by patients with long-COVID and, if confirmed, suggests possible approaches to treatment. It would be ironic if the socio-economic devastation of COVID-19, by intensifying world-wide research in a viral pandemic, leads to valuable insights into other conditions such as ME/CFS, as well as providing additional clues to the aetiology of memory disorders and dementia, including Alzheimer's disease.

https://www.ncbi.nlm.nih.gov/pmc/articles/PMC7890339/

The role of vitamin B12 in viral infections: a comprehensive review of its relationship with the muscle-gut-brain axis and implications for SARS-CoV-2 infection...This comprehensive review establishes the role of vitamin B12 as adjunct therapy for viral infections in the treatment and persistent symptoms of COVID-19, focusing on symptoms related to the muscle-gut-brain axis. Vitamin B12 can help balance immune responses to better fight viral infections. Furthermore, data from randomized clinical trials and meta-analysis indicate that vitamin B12 in the forms of methylcobalamin and cyanocobalamin may increase serum vitamin B12 levels, and resulted in decreased serum methylmalonic acid and homocysteine concentrations, and decreased pain intensity, memory loss, and impaired concentration. Among studies, there is much variation in vitamin B12 doses, chemical forms, supplementation time, and administration routes. Larger randomized clinical trials of vitamin B12 supplementation and analysis of markers such as total vitamin B12, holotranscobalamin, total homocysteine and methylmalonic acid, total folic acid, and, if possible, polymorphisms and methylation of genes need to be conducted with people with and without COVID-19 or who have had COVID-19 to facilitate the proper vitamin B12 form to be administered in individual treatment.

https://pubmed.ncbi.nlm.nih.gov/34791425/

COVID-19 and One-Carbon Metabolism...Dysregulation of one-carbon metabolism affects a wide range of biological processes and is associated with a number of diseases, including cardiovascular disease, dementia, neural tube defects, and cancer. Accumulating evidence suggests that one-carbon metabolism plays an important role in COVID-19. The symptoms of long COVID-19 are similar to those presented by subjects suffering from vitamin B12 deficiency (pernicious anemia). The metabolism of a cell infected by the SARS-CoV-2 virus is reshaped to fulfill the need for massive viral RNA synthesis, which requires de novo purine biosynthesis involving folate and one-carbon metabolism. Many aspects of host sulfur amino acid metabolism, particularly glutathione metabolism underlying antioxidant defenses, are also taken over by the SARS-CoV-2 virus. The purpose of this review is to summarize recent findings related to one-carbon metabolism and sulfur metabolites in COVID-19 and discuss how they inform strategies to combat the disease.

https://pubmed.ncbi.nlm.nih.gov/35456998/

"Prolonged high dosing of vitamin B12 caused a mental awakening in me."

Steven Magee

Vitamin C

Feasibility of Vitamin C in the Treatment of Post Viral Fatigue with Focus on Long COVID, Based on a Systematic Review of IV Vitamin C on Fatigue...Fatigue is common not only in cancer patients but also after viral and other infections. Effective treatment options are still very rare. Therefore, the present knowledge on the pathophysiology of fatigue and the potential positive impact of treatment with vitamin C is illustrated. Additionally, the effectiveness of high-dose IV vitamin C in fatigue resulting from various diseases was assessed by a systematic literature review in order to assess the feasibility of vitamin C in post-viral, especially in long COVID, fatigue. Nine clinical studies with 720 participants were identified. Three of the four controlled trials observed a significant decrease in fatigue scores in the vitamin C group compared to the control group. Four of the five observational or before-and-after studies observed a significant reduction in pre-post levels of fatigue. Attendant symptoms of fatigue such as sleep disturbances, lack of concentration, depression, and pain were also frequently alleviated. Oxidative stress, inflammation, and circulatory disorders, which are important contributors to fatigue, are also discussed in long COVID fatigue. Thus, the antioxidant, anti-inflammatory, endothelial-restoring, and immunomodulatory effects of high-dose IV vitamin C might be a suitable treatment option.

https://pubmed.ncbi.nlm.nih.gov/33807280/

Combining L-Arginine with vitamin C improves long-COVID symptoms: The LINCOLN Survey...Recent evidence suggests that oxidative stress and endothelial dysfunction play critical roles in the pathophysiology of COVID-19 and Long-COVID. We hypothesized that a supplementation combining L-Arginine (to improve endothelial function) and Vitamin C (to reduce oxidation) could have favorable effects on Long-COVID symptoms...supplementation with L-Arginine + Vitamin C has

beneficial effects in Long-COVID, in terms of attenuating its typical symptoms and improving effort perception.
https://pubmed.ncbi.nlm.nih.gov/35868478/

Effects of l-Arginine Plus Vitamin C Supplementation on l-Arginine Metabolism in Adults with Long COVID: Secondary Analysis of a Randomized Clinical Trial...Altered l-arginine metabolism has been described in patients with COVID-19 and has been associated with immune and vascular dysfunction. In the present investigation, we determined the serum concentrations of l-arginine, citrulline, ornithine, monomethyl-l-arginine (MMA), and symmetric and asymmetric dimethylarginine (SDMA, ADMA) in adults with long COVID at baseline and after 28-days of l-arginine plus vitamin C or placebo supplementation enrolled in a randomized clinical trial, compared with a group of adults without previous history of SARS-CoV-2-infection. l-arginine-derived markers of nitric oxide (NO) bioavailability (i.e., l-arginine/ADMA, l-arginine/citrulline+ornithine, and l-arginine/ornithine) were also assayed. Partial least squares discriminant analysis (PLS-DA) models were built to characterize systemic l-arginine metabolism and assess the effects of the supplementation. PLS-DA allowed discrimination of participants with long COVID from healthy controls with 80.2 ± 3.0% accuracy. Lower markers of NO bioavailability were found in participants with long COVID. After 28 days of l-arginine plus vitamin C supplementation, serum l-arginine concentrations and l-arginine/ADMA increased significantly compared with placebo. This supplement may therefore be proposed as a remedy to increase NO bioavailability in people with long COVID.
https://pubmed.ncbi.nlm.nih.gov/36982151/

"Combining vitamin C with other supplements improves its effectiveness."
Steven Magee

Vitamin D

Vitamin D: A Role Also in Long COVID-19?...Vitamin D is an immunomodulatory hormone with proven efficacy against various upper respiratory tract infections. Vitamin D can inhibit hyperinflammatory reactions and accelerate the healing process in the affected areas, especially in lung tissue. Moreover, vitamin D deficiency has been associated with the severity and mortality of COVID-19 cases, with a high prevalence of hypovitaminosis D found in patients with COVID-19 and acute respiratory failure. Thus, there are promising reasons to promote research into the effects of vitamin D supplementation in COVID-19 patients. However, no studies to date have found that vitamin D affects post-COVID-19 symptoms or biomarkers. Based on this scenario, this review aims to provide an up-to-date overview of the potential role of vitamin D in long COVID-19 and of the current literature on this topic.

https://pubmed.ncbi.nlm.nih.gov/35458189/

Low vitamin D levels are associated with Long COVID syndrome in COVID-19 survivors...COVID-19 survivors with Long-COVID have lower 25(OH)vitamin D levels as compared to matched-patients without Long-COVID. Our data suggest that vitamin D levels should be evaluated in COVID-19 patients after hospital-discharge. Role of vitamin D supplementation as preventive strategy of COVID-19 sequelae should be tested in randomized-controlled trials.

https://pubmed.ncbi.nlm.nih.gov/37051747/

A Narrative Review on the Potential Role of Vitamin D3 in the Prevention, Protection, and Disease Mitigation of Acute and Long COVID-19...Epidemiological studies have shown that individuals who were deficient in vitamin D3 had worse COVID-19 health outcomes and mortality rates. Higher doses of vitamin D3 supplementation may improve health and survivorship in individuals of various age groups, comorbidities, and severity of disease symptoms. Vitamin D3's biological effects can provide protection and repair in multiple organ systems affected by SARS-CoV-2. Vitamin D3 supplementation can potentially support disease-mitigation in acute and long COVID-19.

https://pubmed.ncbi.nlm.nih.gov/37145350/

"Long term supplementation with high doses of Vitamin D significantly improved my mental functioning."

Steven Magee

Vitamin E

Dietary Supplements in the Time of COVID-19...many individuals who have had COVID-19 report symptoms of "long COVID" (including breathlessness, cough, fatigue, muscle aches and weakness, sleep difficulties, and cognitive dysfunction) for several weeks, months, or longer after the acute stage of illness has passed. Risk of long COVID appears to be higher in people who are hospitalized following SARS-CoV-2 infection, as well as those who are not vaccinated against COVID-19...Vitamin E is an antioxidant that plays an important role in immune function by helping to maintain cell membrane integrity and by enhancing antibody production, lymphocyte proliferation, and natural killer cell activity. Vitamin E has also been shown to limit inflammation by inhibiting the production of pro-inflammatory cytokines. Vitamin E deficiency impairs both humoral and cell-mediated immunity and increases susceptibility to infections. Some studies suggest that high-dose vitamin E supplements (60 to 800 mg/day) for 1 to 8 months enhance lymphocyte proliferation, interleukin-2 production, and natural killer cell activity in adults aged 60 or older. Frank vitamin E deficiency is rare, except in individuals with intestinal malabsorption disorders. For this reason, research on the ability of vitamin E to improve immune function tends to use supplemental vitamin E rather than simply ensuring that study participants achieve adequate vitamin E status...In one clinical trial, 90 mg (200 IU) vitamin E supplements (as DL-alpha-tocopherol) daily for 1 year reduced the risk of upper respiratory tract infections by 16%, particularly the common cold, in 617 adults aged 65 or older but not lower respiratory tract infections. Supplementation with 50 mg/day vitamin E (as DL-alpha tocopheryl acetate) for 5–8 years also reduced the risk of pneumonia by 69% in 2,216 men aged 50–69 years who smoked 5–19 cigarettes per day and exercised, but it did not affect the risk of pneumonia in another 5,253 men who smoked more than 19 cigarettes per day or did not exercise...because of its effects on immune function, many researchers recommend studying vitamin

E to see if it reduces the risk of COVID-19 or reduces symptoms of the disease...A small clinical trial in Mexico examined the effects of 800 mg vitamin E (as alpha-tocopheryl acetate) every 12 hours for 5 days plus the drug pentoxifylline in 22 hospitalized adults (mean age 57.9 years) with pneumonia that resulted from COVID-19. Another group of 22 patients received pentoxifylline alone. Patients who received vitamin E and pentoxifylline had significantly lower levels of the inflammatory markers interleukin-6 and procalcitonin than at baseline, whereas those who received pentoxifylline alone did not. Vitamin E plus pentoxifylline also significantly decreased the lipid peroxidation index (a measure of oxidative stress), but pentoxifylline alone did not. Both treatments significantly increased nitrite levels (suggesting higher oxygen levels) and reduced levels of the inflammatory marker C-reactive protein, but neither treatment affected total antioxidant capacity.

https://ods.od.nih.gov/factsheets/COVID19-HealthProfessional/

"Vitamin E increases nitrate levels in the body that are linked to higher oxygen levels."

Steven Magee

Calcium

A Google search of 'calcium pubmed 2023 long covid' produced no relevant findings. It appears there is little research being done in this area.

"COVID-19 is associated with low calcium."

Steven Magee

Iron

The Impact of Iron Dyshomeostasis and Anaemia on Long-Term Pulmonary Recovery and Persisting Symptom Burden after COVID-19: A Prospective Observational Cohort Study

...Coronavirus disease 2019 (COVID-19) is frequently associated with iron dyshomeostasis. The latter is related to acute disease severity and COVID-19 convalescence...At 60 days post-COVID-19 follow-up, hyperferritinaemia (35% of patients), iron deficiency (24% of the cohort) and anaemia (9% of the patients) were frequently found. Anaemia of inflammation (AI) was the predominant feature at early post-acute follow-up, whereas the anaemia phenotype shifted towards iron deficiency anaemia (IDA) and combinations of IDA and AI until the 360 days follow-up. The prevalence of anaemia significantly decreased over time, but iron dyshomeostasis remained a frequent finding throughout the study. Neither iron dyshomeostasis nor anaemia were related to persisting structural lung impairment, but both were associated with impaired stress resilience at long-term COVID-19 follow-up. To conclude, iron dyshomeostasis and anaemia are frequent findings after COVID-19 and may contribute to its long-term symptomatic outcome.

https://www.ncbi.nlm.nih.gov/pmc/articles/PMC9228477/

SARS-CoV-2 Infection Dysregulates Host Iron (Fe)-Redox Homeostasis (Fe-R-H): Role of Fe-Redox Regulators, Ferroptosis Inhibitors, Anticoagulants, and Iron-Chelators in COVID-19 Control

...Severe imbalance in iron metabolism among SARS-CoV-2 infected patients is prominent in every symptomatic (mild, moderate to severe) clinical phase of COVID-19. Phase-I - Hypoxia correlates with reduced O2 transport by erythrocytes, overexpression of HIF-1α, altered mitochondrial bioenergetics with host metabolic reprogramming (HMR). Phase-II - Hyperferritinemia results from an increased iron overload, which triggers a fulminant proinflammatory response - the acute cytokine release syndrome (CRS). Elevated cytokine levels (i.e. IL6, TNFα and CRP) strongly correlates with altered ferritin/TF ratios in COVID-19 patients. Phase-III - Thromboembolism is consequential to erythrocyte dysfunction with heme release, increased prothrombin time and elevated D-dimers, cumulatively linked to severe coagulopathies with life-threatening outcomes such as ARDS, and multi-organ failure. Taken together, Fe-R-H dysregulation is implicated in every symptomatic phase of COVID-19. Fe-R-H regulators such as lactoferrin (LF), hemoxygenase-1 (HO-1), erythropoietin (EPO) and hepcidin modulators are innate bio-replenishments that sequester iron, neutralize iron-mediated free radicals, reduce oxidative stress, and improve host defense by optimizing iron metabolism. Due to its pivotal role in 'cytokine storm', ferroptosis is a potential intervention target. Ferroptosis inhibitors such as ferrostatin-1, liproxstatin-1, quercetin, and melatonin could prevent mitochondrial lipid peroxidation, up-regulate antioxidant/GSH levels and abrogate iron overload-induced apoptosis through activation of Nrf2 and HO-1 signaling pathways. Iron chelators such as heparin, deferoxamine, caffeic acid, curcumin, α-lipoic acid, and phytic acid could protect against ferroptosis and restore mitochondrial function, iron-redox potential, and rebalance Fe-R-H status. Therefore, Fe-R-H restoration is a host biomarker-driven potential combat strategy for an effective clinical and post-recovery management of COVID-19.

https://pubmed.ncbi.nlm.nih.gov/35603834/

"Iron imbalance is a feature of COVID-19."

Steven Magee

Magnesium

The relevance of magnesium homeostasis in COVID-19...

existing data seem to corroborate an association between deranged magnesium homeostasis and COVID-19, and call for further and better studies to explore the prophylactic or therapeutic potential of magnesium supplementation...We propose to reconsider the relevance of magnesium, frequently overlooked in clinical practice. Therefore, magnesemia should be monitored and, in case of imbalanced magnesium homeostasis, an appropriate nutritional regimen or supplementation might contribute to protect against SARS-CoV-2 infection, reduce severity of COVID-19 symptoms and facilitate the recovery after the acute phase...evidence is accumulating about the lingering effects experienced by recovered COVID-19 patients, even after a mild to moderate disease. While scientists are searching for a specific therapy to treat the disease, there is an urgent need to individuate strategies to reinforce the immune system and prevent the infection, to mitigate the progression of the disease, and to ameliorate symptoms of long COVID. A balanced diet is essential to strengthen immune responses and to harmonize the microbiota, a complex ecosystem important for health. The nutritional status of the patient influences the course of COVID-19, however knowledge about the nutritional support of COVID patients is very limited...it is noteworthy that in the brain magnesium affects multiple biochemical processes involved in cognitive functions, cell membrane stability and integrity, NMDA-receptor response to excitatory stimuli. It also exerts a calcium-antagonist action and combats neuroinflammation. Consistently, magnesium deficit determines anxiety, insomnia, hyperemotionality, depression, headache, light-headedness, symptoms included in the post-acute COVID-19 syndrome. Moreover, magnesium deficits have been suggested to cause weakness and muscle pain. This is not surprising since magnesium is key for all the enzymes utilizing or synthesizing muscle ATP, and thus for the production of muscle energy, and also regulates contraction and relaxation. Additionally, magnesium assures the regenerative capacity of skeletal muscle fibers. In conclusion, an altered magnesium homeostasis might reasonably contribute to and aggravate long COVID syndrome. Therefore, assessing and, if necessary, correcting magnesaemia is essential to support full recovery. It is clear that care for patients with COVID-19 does not end at the time of hospital discharge, and comprehensive care of recovered patients is needed in the outpatient setting as well. In this respect, magnesium supplementation is a safe and cost-effective intervention that could help restoring the severely deranged homeostatic equilibrium of the body.

https://www.ncbi.nlm.nih.gov/pmc/articles/PMC8540865/

Prognostic Value of Magnesium in COVID-19: Findings from the COMEPA Study...Magnesium (Mg) plays a key role in infections. However, its role in coronavirus disease 2019 (COVID-19) is still underexplored, particularly in long-term sequelae. The aim of the present study was to examine the prognostic value of serum Mg levels in older people affected by COVID-19. Patients were divided into those with serum Mg levels ≤1.96 vs. >1.96 mg/dL, according to the Youden index. A total of 260 participants (mean age 65 years, 53.8% males) had valid Mg measurements. Serum Mg had a good accuracy in predicting in-hospital mortality (area under the curve = 0.83; 95% CI: 0.74-0.91). Low serum Mg at admission significantly predicted in-hospital death (HR = 1.29; 95% CI: 1.03-2.68) after adjusting for several confounders. A value of Mg ≤ 1.96 mg/dL was associated with a longer mean length of stay compared to those with a serum Mg > 1.96 (15.2 vs. 12.7 days). Low serum Mg was associated with a higher incidence of long COVID symptomatology (OR = 2.14; 95% CI: 1.30-4.31), particularly post-traumatic stress disorder (OR = 2.00; 95% CI: 1.24-16.40). In conclusion, low serum Mg levels were significant predictors of mortality, length of stay, and onset of long COVID symptoms, indicating that measuring serum Mg in COVID-19 may be helpful in the prediction of complications related to the disease.

https://pubmed.ncbi.nlm.nih.gov/36839188/

"Magnesium is a known treatment for Long COVID."

Steven Magee

Zinc

Nutritional deficiencies that may predispose to long COVID...Multiple nutritional deficiencies (MND) confound studies designed to assess the role of a single nutrient in contributing to the initiation and progression of disease states. Despite the perception of many healthcare practitioners, up to 25% of Americans are deficient in five-or-more essential nutrients. Stress associated with the COVID-19 pandemic further increases the prevalence of deficiency states. Viral infections compete for crucial nutrients with immune cells. Viral replication and proliferation of immunocompetent cells critical to the host response require these essential nutrients, including zinc. Clinical studies have linked levels of more than 22 different dietary components to the likelihood of COVID-19 infection and the severity of the disease. People at higher risk of infection due to MND are also more likely to have long-term sequelae, known as Long COVID.

https://pubmed.ncbi.nlm.nih.gov/36920723/

Symptom Profile of Patients With Post-COVID-19 Conditions and Influencing Factors for Recovery...Background: The aim of the study was to examine the factors that influence the improvement of post-coronavirus disease 2019 (COVID-19) symptoms. Methods: We investigated the biomarkers and post-COVID-19 symptoms status of 120 post-COVID-19 symptomatic outpatients (44 males and 76 females) visiting our hospital. This study was a retrospective analysis, so we analyzed the course of symptoms only for those who could follow the progress of the symptoms for 12 weeks. We analyzed the data including the intake of zinc acetate hydrate. Results: The main symptoms that remained after 12 weeks were, in descending order: taste disorder, olfactory disorder, hair loss, and fatigue. Fatigue was improved in all cases treated with zinc acetate hydrate 8 weeks later, exhibiting a significant difference from the untreated group

(P = 0.030). The similar trend was observed even 12 weeks later, although there was no significant difference (P = 0.060). With respect to hair loss, the group treated with zinc acetate hydrate showed significant improvements 4, 8, and 12 weeks later, compared with the untreated group (P = 0.002, P = 0.002, and P = 0.006). Conclusion: Zinc acetate hydrate may improve fatigue and hair loss as symptoms after contracting COVID-19.

https://www.ncbi.nlm.nih.gov/pmc/articles/PMC9990724/

Symptomatic Characteristics of Hypozincemia Detected in Long COVID Patients...Objectives: The aim of this study was to determine the characteristics of hypozincemia in long COVID patients. Methods: This study was a single-center retrospective observational study for outpatients who visited the long COVID clinic established in a university hospital during the period from 15 February 2021 to 28 February 2022. Characteristics of patients with a serum zinc concentration lower than 70 μg/dL (10.7 μmol/L) were compared with characteristics of patients with normozincemia. Results: In a total of 194 patients with long COVID after excluding 32 patients, hypozincemia was detected in 43 patients (22.2%) including 16 male patients (37.2%) and 27 female patients (62.8%). Among various parameters including the background characteristics of the patients and medical histories, the patients with hypozincemia were significantly older than the patients with normozincemia (median age: 50 vs. 39 years). A significant negative correlation was found between serum zinc concentrations and age in male patients (R = -0.39; p < 0.01) but not in female patients. In addition, there was no significant correlation between serum zinc levels and inflammatory markers. General fatigue was the most frequent symptom in both male patients with hypozincemia (9 out of 16: 56.3%) and female patients with hypozincemia (8 out of 27: 29.6%). Patients with severe hypozincemia (serum zinc level lower than 60 μg/dL) had major complaints of dysosmia and dysgeusia, which were more frequent complaints than general fatigue. Conclusions: The most frequent symptom in long COVID patients with hypozincemia was general fatigue. Serum zinc levels should be measured in long COVID patients with general fatigue, particularly in male patients. https://pubmed.ncbi.nlm.nih.gov/36902849/

Long-COVID post-viral chronic fatigue and affective symptoms are associated with oxidative damage, lowered antioxidant defenses and inflammation: a proof of concept and mechanism study...The immune-inflammatory response during the acute phase of COVID-19, as assessed using peak body temperature (PBT) and peripheral oxygen saturation (SpO2), predicts the severity of chronic fatigue, depression and anxiety symptoms 3-4 months later. The present study was performed to examine the effects of SpO2 and PBT during acute infection on immune, oxidative and nitrosative stress (IO&NS) pathways and neuropsychiatric symptoms of Long COVID. This study assayed SpO2 and PBT during acute COVID-19, and C-reactive protein (CRP), malondialdehyde (MDA), protein carbonyls (PCs), myeloperoxidase (MPO), nitric oxide (NO), zinc, and glutathione peroxidase (Gpx) in 120 Long COVID individuals and 36 controls. Cluster analysis showed that 31.7% of the Long COVID patients had severe abnormalities in SpO2, body temperature, increased oxidative toxicity (OSTOX) and lowered antioxidant defenses (ANTIOX), and increased total Hamilton Depression (HAMD) and Anxiety (HAMA) and Fibromylagia-Fatigue (FF) scores. Around 60% of the variance in the neuropsychiatric symptoms of Long COVID (a factor extracted from HAMD, HAMA and FF scores) was explained by OSTOX/ANTIOX ratio, PBT and SpO2. Increased PBT predicted increased CRP and lowered ANTIOX and zinc levels, while lowered SpO2 predicted lowered Gpx and increased NO production. Lowered SpO2 strongly predicts OSTOX/ANTIOX during Long COVID. In conclusion, the impact of acute COVID-19 on the symptoms of Long COVID is partly mediated by OSTOX/ANTIOX, especially lowered Gpx and zinc, increased MPO and NO production and lipid peroxidation-associated aldehyde formation. The results suggest that post-viral somatic and mental symptoms have a neuroimmune and neuro-oxidative origin.

https://pubmed.ncbi.nlm.nih.gov/36280755/

"Zinc supplementation is a common treatment for Long COVID."

Steven Magee

Alpha Lipoic Acid (ALA)

Nutritional Support During Long COVID: A Systematic Scoping Review...Introduction: Long COVID is a term that encompasses a range of signs, symptoms, and sequalae that continue or develop after an acute COVID-19 infection. The lack of early recognition of the condition contributed to delays in identifying factors that may contribute toward its development and prevention. The aim of this study was to scope the available literature to identify potential nutritional interventions to support people with symptoms associated with long COVID. Methods: This study was designed as a systematic scoping review of the literature (registration PROSPERO CRD42022306051). Studies with participants aged 18 years or older, with long COVID and who underwent a nutritional intervention were included in the review. Results: A total of 285 citations were initially identified, with five papers eligible for inclusion: two were pilot studies of nutritional supplements in the community, and three were nutritional interventions as part of inpatient or outpatient multidisciplinary rehabilitation programs. There were two broad categories of interventions: those that focused on compositions of nutrients (including micronutrients such as vitamin and mineral supplements) and those that were incorporated as part of multidisciplinary rehabilitation programs. Nutrients included in more than one study were multiple B group vitamins, vitamin C, vitamin D, and acetyl-l-carnitine. Discussion: Two studies trialed nutritional supplements for long COVID in community samples. Although these initial reports were positive, they are based on poorly designed studies and therefore cannot provide conclusive evidence. Nutritional rehabilitation was an important aspect of recovery from severe inflammation, malnutrition, and sarcopenia in hospital rehabilitation programs. Current gaps in the literature include a potential role for anti-inflammatory nutrients such as the omega 3 fatty acids, which are currently undergoing clinical trials, glutathione-boosting treatments such as N-acetylcysteine, alpha-lipoic acid, or liposomal glutathione in long COVID, and a possible adjunctive role for anti-inflammatory dietary interventions. This review provides preliminary evidence that nutritional interventions may be an important part of a rehabilitation program for people with severe long COVID symptomatology, including severe inflammation, malnutrition, and sarcopenia. For those in the general population with long COVID symptoms, the role of specific nutrients has not yet been studied well enough to recommend any particular nutrient or dietary intervention as a treatment or adjunctive treatment. Clinical trials of single nutrients are currently being conducted, and future systematic reviews could focus on single nutrient or dietary interventions to identify their nuanced mechanisms of action. Further clinical studies incorporating complex nutritional interventions are also warranted to strengthen the evidence base for using nutrition as a useful adjunctive treatment for people living with long COVID.

https://pubmed.ncbi.nlm.nih.gov/37102680/

Coenzyme Q10 + alpha lipoic acid for chronic COVID syndrome...Chronic COVID syndrome is characterized by chronic fatigue, myalgia, depression and sleep disturbances, similar to chronic fatigue syndrome (CFS) and fibromyalgia syndrome. Implementations of mitochondrial nutrients (MNs) with diet are important for the clinical effects antioxidant. We examined if use of an association of coenzyme Q10 and alpha lipoic acid (Requpero®) could reduce chronic covid symptoms. The Requpero study is a prospective observational study in which 174 patients, who had developed chronic-covid syndrome, were divided in two groups: The first one (116 patients) received coenzyme Q10 + alpha lipoic acid, and the second one (58 patients) did not receive any treatment. Primary outcome was reduction in Fatigue Severity Scale (FSS) in treatment group compared with control group. Complete FSS response was reached most frequently in treatment group than in control group. A FSS complete response was reached in 62 (53.5%) patients in treatment group and in two (3.5%) patients in control group. A reduction in FSS core < 20% from baseline at T1 (non-response) was observed in 11 patients in the treatment group (9.5%) and in 15 patients in the control group

(25.9%) (p < 0.0001). To date, this is the first study that tests the efficacy of coenzyme Q10 and alpha lipoic acid in chronic Covid syndrome. Primary and secondary outcomes were met. These results have to be confirmed through a double blind placebo controlled trial of longer duration.

https://pubmed.ncbi.nlm.nih.gov/35994177/

Neurological and Neuromuscular Sequelae of COVID-19...there is a growing body of evidence that post-acute sequelae of SARS-CoV-2 infection (PASC) can manifest as neurologic sequelae...Alpha lipoic acid, often an over the counter antioxidant and insulin-memetic supplement, can be prescribed at 600mg daily for smell dysfunction associated with viral infections, and it is in this author's experience that it has been effective when paired with smell therapy in treating post-COVID anosmia, but it can take at least 3 months of medication administration before effect and further research is still needed to establish more definitive efficacy. However, recently some providers have noticed an increasing number of case reports evidence of neural epidermal growth factor-like 1 (NELL1) associated glomerulonephritis linked to alpha lipoic acid administration, with acute presentation of proteinuria and acute nephrotic syndrome that resolved with medication cessation. Though still relatively rare and more studies are needed for formal guidelines to be established, consideration of checking for proteinuria and hypoalbuminemia may be indicated should a patient develop acute onset edema.

https://www.ncbi.nlm.nih.gov/pmc/articles/PMC10076508/

Towards a Better Understanding of the Complexities of Myalgic Encephalomyelitis/Chronic Fatigue Syndrome and Long COVID...The 'ME/CFS-like' Long COVID patients suffering from the post viral fatigue syndrome have a single originating stressor, the SARS-CoV-2 virus. They provide a unique opportunity to evaluate whether subtypes might arise from different initiators. Long COVID has some unique characteristics that apparently relate to the specific SARS-CoV-2 virus, such as the loss of taste and smell, and conditions such as enhanced skin problems, a loss of voice control, and breathlessness in some of those affected. However, most of the many symptoms ascribed to ME/CFS have also been associated with Long COVID (and are also found in only a proportion of the cases in this cohort). This would indicate there are multiple phenotypes among Long COVID patients as well, and indeed analysis of health record data from two large patient cohorts has identified four subtypes...Currently, there is a dearth of therapeutic options for ME/CFS patients and promising treatments have rarely resulted in validating trials that enable more comprehensive studies. When a promising treatment does not benefit most patients, impetus for further studies is often lost. Since combinations of treatments might be beneficial, trials of a promising candidate therapeutic in combination with other compounds are needed. There are examples of small studies with such combinations that are indeed showing promise, including CoQ10 and Se and CoQ10 and lipoic acid.

https://www.ncbi.nlm.nih.gov/pmc/articles/PMC10048882/

"Alpha Lipoic Acid is emerging as a treatment for Long COVID."

Steven Magee

Female Hormones

Long COVID: an estrogen-associated autoimmune disease?...No abstract available.

https://pubmed.ncbi.nlm.nih.gov/33850105/

"Hormone dysfunction is a feature of Long COVID."

Steven Magee

Male Hormones

Testosterone in males with COVID-19: A 7-month cohort study...Circulating testosterone levels have been found to be reduced in men with severe acute respiratory syndrome coronavirus 2 infection, COVID-19, with lower levels being associated with more severe clinical outcomes...Although total testosterone levels increased over time after COVID-19, more than 50% of men who recovered from the disease still had circulating testosterone levels suggestive for a condition of hypogonadism at 7-month follow-up. In as many as 10% of cases, testosterone levels even further decreased. Of clinical relevance, the higher the burden of comorbid conditions at presentation, the lower the probability of testosterone levels recovery over time.

https://pubmed.ncbi.nlm.nih.gov/34409772/

Testosterone and Covid-19: An update...There is overwhelming evidence to suggest that male gender is at a higher risk of developing more severe Covid-19 disease and thus having poorer clinical outcomes...the evidence so far suggests that the role of testosterone in Covid-19 is a double-edged sword, with some studies suggesting that a low testosterone state is protective in men in certain situations, yet increasing amounts of evidence suggests lower T in male patients is associated with increased Covid-19 severity and mortality. However, lack of evidence on the effect of pre-infection circulating T, contradictory reports on the effects of ADT on SAR-CoV-2 infection, and incomplete understanding of the underlying biological mechanisms makes it difficult to conclude if T is a marker or mediator of Covid-19 severity. Indeed, the mechanisms are likely to be multidimensional and influenced by a wide range of interacting factors that can be specific to the individual patient. Furthermore, the potential of TTh in men with Covid-19 to aid recovery and the effect of testosterone on long Covid are still to be extensively investigated.

https://www.ncbi.nlm.nih.gov/pmc/articles/PMC9537909/

Testosterone in males with COVID-19: a 12-month cohort study...Male patients with COVID-19 have been found with reduced serum total testosterone (tT) levels and with more severe clinical outcomes...Circulating tT levels keep increasing over time in men after COVID-19. Still, almost 30% of men who recovered from COVID-19 had low circulating T levels suggestive for a condition of hypogonadism at a minimum 12-month follow-up.

https://pubmed.ncbi.nlm.nih.gov/36251583/

Detection of Male Hypogonadism in Patients with Post COVID-19 Condition...The pathogenesis and prognosis of post COVID-19 condition have remained unclear. We set up an outpatient clinic specializing in long COVID in February 2021 and we have been investigating post COVID-19 condition. Based on the results of our earlier study showing that "general fatigue" mimicking myalgic encephalomyelitis/chronic fatigue syndrome (ME/CFS) is the most common symptom in long COVID patients, a retrospective analysis was performed for 39 male patients in whom serum free testosterone (FT) levels were measured out of 61 male patients who visited our clinic. We analyzed the medical records of the patients' backgrounds, symptoms and laboratory results. Among the 39 patients, 19 patients (48.7%) met the criteria for late-onset hypogonadism (LOH; FT < 8.5 pg/mL: LOH group) and 14 patients were under 50 years of age. A weak negative correlation was found between age and serum FT level ($r = -0.301$, $p = 0.0624$). Symptoms including general fatigue, anxiety, cough and hair loss were more frequent in the LOH group than in the non-LOH group (FT $\geq$ 8.5 pg/mL). Among various laboratory parameters, blood hemoglobin level was slightly, but significantly, lower in the LOH group. Serum level of FT was positively correlated with the levels of blood hemoglobin and serum total protein and albumin in the total population, whereas these interrelationships were blurred in the

LOH group. Collectively, the results indicate that the incidence of LOH is relatively high in male patients, even young male patients, with post COVID-19 and that serum FT measurement is useful for revealing occult LOH status in patients with long COVID.

https://pubmed.ncbi.nlm.nih.gov/35407562/

Long COVID and risk of erectile dysfunction in recovered patients from mild to moderate COVID-19...Patients with coronavirus disease 2019 (COVID-19) were shown to have reduced serum testosterone levels compared to healthy individuals. Low testosterone levels are linked with the development of erectile dysfunction (ED). In this case-controlled study, 20 healthy controls and 39 patients with ED 3 months after recovering from mild-to-moderate COVID-19 pneumonia were studied. The patients ranged in age from 31 to 47 years. To identify early and late COVID-19 infections, real-time polymerase-chain reaction (RT-PCR) and COVID-19 antibody testing were done. The levels of luteinizing hormone (LH), follicular stimulating hormone (FSH), total testosterone (TT), free testosterone (FT), free androgenic index (FAI), and sex hormone-binding globulin (SHBG) were measured. The sexual health inventory for patients (SHIM) score was used to measure the erectile function of the patients and controls. When compared to the controls, the TT serum level in long COVID-19 (LC) patients with ED was low ($p = 0.01$). In contrast to controls, FT and FAI were both lower in LC patients with ED. ($p = 0.001$). FSH serum levels did not significantly differ ($p = 0.07$), but in ED patients, LH serum levels were elevated. SHIM scores were associated with low TT ($p = 0.30$), FT ($p = 0.09$), and high LH ($p = 0.76$) in LC patients with ED. Male patients with decreased serum levels of LH and testosterone may have hypothalamic-pituitary-gonadal axis dysfunction, which could lead to the development of LC-induced ED. Therefore, an in-depth research is necessary to confirm the causal link between COVID-19 and ED in LC patients.

https://pubmed.ncbi.nlm.nih.gov/37045862/

SARS-CoV-2 and male infertility: from short- to long-term impacts...Purpose: The coronavirus 2019 (COVID-19) pandemic-caused by a new type of severe acute respiratory syndrome coronavirus 2 (SARS-CoV-2)-has posed severe impacts on public health worldwide and has resulted in a total of > 6 million deaths. Notably, male patients developed more complications and had mortality rates ~ 77% higher than those of female patients. The extensive expression of the SARS-CoV-2 receptor and related proteins in the male reproductive tract and the association of serum testosterone levels with viral entry and infection have brought attention to COVID-19's effects on male fertility. Methods: The peer-reviewed articles and reviews were obtained by searching for the keywords SARS-CoV-2, COVID-19, endocrine, spermatogenesis, epididymis, prostate, and vaccine in the databases of PubMed, Web of Science and Google Scholar from 2020-2022. Results: This review summarizes the effects of COVID-19 on male reproductive system and investigates the impact of various types of SARS-CoV-2 vaccines on male reproductive health. We also present the underlying mechanisms by which SARS-CoV-2 affects male reproduction and discuss the potentially harmful effects of asymptomatic infections, as well as the long-term impact of COVID-19 on male reproductive health. Conclusion: COVID-19 disrupted the HPG axis, which had negative impacts on spermatogenesis and the epididymis, albeit further investigations need to be performed. The development of vaccines against various SARS-CoV-2 variations is important to lower infection rates and long-term COVID risks.

https://pubmed.ncbi.nlm.nih.gov/36917421/

"Long COVID is associated with lowered testosterone levels."

Steven Magee

Fish Oil Supplements

Long COVID and long chain fatty acids (LCFAs): Psychoneuroimmunity implication of omega-3 LCFAs in delayed consequences of COVID-19... The global spread of severe acute respiratory syndrome coronavirus 2 (SARS-CoV-2) has led to the lasting pandemic of coronavirus disease 2019 (COVID-19) and the post-acute phase sequelae of heterogeneous negative impacts in multiple systems known as the "long COVID." The mechanisms of neuropsychiatric complications of long COVID are multifactorial, including long-term tissue damages from direct CNS viral involvement, unresolved systemic inflammation and oxidative stress, maladaptation of the renin-angiotensin-aldosterone system and coagulation system, dysregulated immunity, the dysfunction of neurotransmitters and hypothalamus–pituitaryadrenal (HPA) axis, and the psychosocial stress imposed by societal changes in response to this pandemic. The strength of safety, well-acceptance, and accumulating scientific evidence has now afforded nutritional medicine a place in the mainstream of neuropsychiatric intervention and prophylaxis. Long chain omega-3 polyunsaturated fatty acids (omega-3 or n-3 PUFAs) might have favorable effects on immunity, inflammation, oxidative stress and psychoneuroimmunity at different stages of SARS-CoV-2 infection. Omega-3 PUFAs, particularly EPA, have shown effects in treating mood and neurocognitive disorders by reducing pro-inflammatory cytokines, altering the HPA axis, and modulating neurotransmission via lipid rafts. In addition, omega-3 PUFAs and their metabolites, including specialized pro-resolvin mediators, accelerate the process of cleansing chronic inflammation and restoring tissue homeostasis, and therefore offer a promising strategy for Long COVID. In this article, we explore in a systematic review the putative molecular mechanisms by which omega-3 PUFAs and their metabolites counteract the negative effects of long COVID on the brain, behavior, and immunity.

https://www.ncbi.nlm.nih.gov/pmc/articles/PMC8977215/

A multi-omics based anti-inflammatory immune signature characterizes long COVID-19 syndrome...To investigate long COVID-19 syndrome (LCS) pathophysiology, we performed an exploratory study with blood plasma derived from three groups: 1) healthy vaccinated individuals without SARS-CoV-2 exposure; 2) asymptomatic recovered patients at least three months after SARS-CoV-2 infection and; 3) symptomatic patients at least 3 months after SARS-CoV-2 infection with chronic fatigue syndrome or similar symptoms, here designated as patients with long COVID-19 syndrome (LCS). Multiplex cytokine profiling indicated slightly elevated pro-inflammatory cytokine levels in recovered individuals in contrast to patients with LCS. Plasma proteomics demonstrated low levels of acute phase proteins and macrophage-derived secreted proteins in LCS. High levels of anti-inflammatory oxylipins including omega-3 fatty acids in LCS were detected by eicosadomics, whereas targeted metabolic profiling indicated high levels of anti-inflammatory osmolytes taurine and hypaphorine, but low amino acid and triglyceride levels and deregulated acylcarnitines. A model considering alternatively polarized macrophages as a major contributor to these molecular alterations is presented.

https://pubmed.ncbi.nlm.nih.gov/36507225/

"Fish oil appears to have a promising role in reducing Long COVID symptoms."

Steven Magee

Live Culture Yogurt

A Google search of 'pubmed 2023 long covid live culture yogurt' produced no relevant findings. It appears there is little research being done in this area.

"I eat live culture yogurt daily to treat my Long COVID symptoms."

Steven Magee

Amino Acids

Long COVID: Is there a kidney link?...Metabolic causes such as altered bioenergetics and amino acid metabolism may play a major role in Long COVID. Renal-metabolic regulation is an integral part of these pathways but has not been systematically or routinely investigated in Long COVID. Here we discuss the biochemistry of renal tubular injury as it may contribute to Long COVID symptoms. We propose three potential mechanisms that could be involved in Long COVID namely creatine phosphate metabolism, un-reclaimed glomerular filtrate and COVID specific proximal tubule cells (PTC) injury-a tryptophan paradigm. This approach is intended to allow for improved diagnostics and therapy for the long-haul sufferers.

https://pubmed.ncbi.nlm.nih.gov/37077670/

"Amino acids were a key ingredient in my recovery from Long COVID symptoms."

Steven Magee

Glycine

A Google search of 'pubmed 2023 long covid glycine' produced no relevant findings. It appears there is little research being done in this area.

"Glycine with carnitine is the foundation of my supplementation protocol for Long COVID symptoms."

Steven Magee

L-Carnitine

Can l-carnitine reduce post-COVID-19 fatigue?...A significant number of patients infected with the new coronavirus suffer from chronic fatigue syndrome after COVID-19, and their symptoms may persist for months after the infection. Nevertheless, no particular treatment for post-disease fatigue has been found. At the same time, many clinical trials have shown the effectiveness of l-carnitine in relieving fatigue caused by the treatment of diseases such as cancer, MS, and many other diseases. Therefore, it can be considered as a potential option to eliminate the effects of fatigue caused by COVID-19, and its consumption is recommended in future clinical trials to evaluate its effectiveness and safety.

https://www.ncbi.nlm.nih.gov/pmc/articles/PMC8667465/

Dietary supplements for the management of COVID-19 symptoms...The aim of this paper is to review the relationship between COVID-19 and nutrition and to discuss to most up-to-date dietary supplements proposed for COVID-19 treatment and prevention. Nutrition and nutritional dysregulations, such as obesity and malnutrition, are prominent risk factors for severe COVID-19. These factors exert anti-inflammatory and proinflammatory effects on the immune system, thus exacerbating or reducing the immunological response against the virus. As for the nutritional habits, the Western diet induces a chronic inflammatory state, whereas the Mediterranean diet exerts anti-inflammatory effects and has been proposed for ameliorating COVID-19 evolution and symptoms. Several vaccines have been researched and commercialized for COVID-19 prevention, whereas several drugs, although clinically tested, have not shown promising effects. To compensate for the lack of treatment, several supplements have been recommended for preventing or ameliorating COVID-19 symptoms. Thus, it is critical to review the dietary supplements proposed for COVID-19 treatment. Supplements containing α-cyclodextrin and hydroxytyrosol exhibited promising effects in several clinical trials and reduced the severity of the outcomes and the duration of the infection. Moreover, a supplement containing hydroxytyrosol, acetyl L-carnitine, and vitamins B, C, and D improved the symptoms of patients with post-COVID syndrome.

https://www.ncbi.nlm.nih.gov/pmc/articles/PMC9710408/

Biomedical role of L-carnitine in several organ systems, cellular tissues, and COVID-19...Carnitine is a conditionally necessary vitamin that aids in energy creation and fatty acid metabolism. Its bioavailability is higher in vegetarians than in meat-eaters. Deficits in carnitine transporters occur because of genetic mutations or in conjunction with other illnesses. Carnitine shortage can arise in health issues and diseases-including hypoglycaemia, heart disease, starvation, cirrhosis, and ageing-because of abnormalities in carnitine control. The physiologically active form of L-carnitine supports immunological function in diabetic patients. Carnitine has been demonstrated to be effective in the treatment of Alzheimer's disease, several painful neuropathies, and other conditions. It has been used as a dietary supplement for the treatment of heart disease, and it also aids in the treatment of obesity and reduces blood glucose levels. Therefore, L-carnitine shows the potential to eliminate the influences of fatigue in COVID-19, and its consumption is recommended in future clinical trials to estimate its efficacy and safety. This review focused on carnitine and its effect on tissues, covering the biosynthesis, metabolism, bioavailability, biological actions, and its effects on various body systems and COVID-19.

https://pubmed.ncbi.nlm.nih.gov/36629544/

"L-Carnitine is commonly used to improve heart health."
Steven Magee

L-Carnitine L-Tartrate

Combined Metabolic Activators Accelerates Recovery in Mild-to-Moderate COVID-19...COVID-19 is associated with mitochondrial dysfunction and metabolic abnormalities, including the deficiencies in nicotinamide adenine dinucleotide (NAD+) and glutathione metabolism. Here it is investigated if administration of a mixture of combined metabolic activators (CMAs) consisting of glutathione and NAD+ precursors can restore metabolic function and thus aid the recovery of COVID-19 patients. CMAs include l-serine, N-acetyl-l-cysteine, nicotinamide riboside, and l-carnitine tartrate, salt form of l-carnitine. Placebo-controlled, open-label phase 2 study and double-blinded phase 3 clinical trials are conducted to investigate the time of symptom-free recovery on ambulatory patients using CMAs. The results of both studies show that the time to complete recovery is significantly shorter in the CMA group (6.6 vs 9.3 d) in phase 2 and (5.7 vs 9.2 d) in phase 3 trials compared to placebo group. A comprehensive analysis of the plasma metabolome and proteome reveals major metabolic changes. Plasma levels of proteins and metabolites associated with inflammation and antioxidant metabolism are significantly improved in patients treated with CMAs as compared to placebo. The results show that treating patients infected with COVID-19 with CMAs lead to a more rapid symptom-free recovery, suggesting a role for such a therapeutic regime in the treatment of infections leading to respiratory problems...l-carnitine is a naturally occurring substance required in mammalian energy metabolism. It is a carrier molecule that facilitates the transport of long-chain fatty acids across the inner mitochondrial membrane, thereby delivering substrate for oxidation and subsequent energy production. l-carnitine has been reported to possess antioxidant and anti-inflammatory potency and its increase might be associated with the relatively decreased inflammatory response in the patients. The results of another study using a lamb model with increased pulmonary blood flow showed that chronic l-carnitine treatment alleviates changes in lung carnitine homeostasis, reduces associated oxidative stress, and improves pulmonary mitochondrial function, NO signaling and eventually endothelial function...Many COVID-19 patients are at risk for detrimental outcomes due to systemic inflammatory responses referred to as a cytokine storm, a life-threatening condition is dependent on downstream processes that lead to oxidative stress, dysregulation of iron homeostasis, hypercoagulability, and thrombocytopenia. Several studies have proposed that CMA components may effectively inhibit the production of proinflammatory molecules (e.g., IL-6, CCL-5, CXCL-8, and CXCL-10) and improve impaired mitochondrial functions by reducing oxidative damage, lipid peroxidation, and disturbed glucose tolerance. Based on integrative analysis, we observed that CMA may interrupt the overactive immune response and early treatment with CMA may reduce the risk of progression to severe respiratory distress and lung damage.

https://www.ncbi.nlm.nih.gov/pmc/articles/PMC8420376/

"I take L-Carnitine L-Tartrate when I cannot obtain L-Carnitine to treat my Long COVID symptoms."

Steven Magee

GPLC

A Google search of 'pubmed 2023 long covid GPLC glycine propionyl l-carnitine' produced no relevant findings. It appears there is little research being done in this area.

"GPLC treats hypoxic altitude sickness."

Steven Magee

L-Arginine

Combining l-Arginine with vitamin C improves long-COVID symptoms: The LINCOLN Survey...Our survey indicates that the supplementation with l-Arginine + Vitamin C has beneficial effects in Long-COVID, in terms of attenuating its typical symptoms and improving effort perception. https://www.ncbi.nlm.nih.gov/pmc/articles/PMC9295384/

Effects of l-Arginine Plus Vitamin C Supplementation on l-Arginine Metabolism in Adults with Long COVID: Secondary Analysis of a Randomized Clinical Trial...Altered l-arginine metabolism has been described in patients with COVID-19 and has been associated with immune and vascular dysfunction. In the present investigation, we determined the serum concentrations of l-arginine, citrulline, ornithine, monomethyl-l-arginine (MMA), and symmetric and asymmetric dimethylarginine (SDMA, ADMA) in adults with long COVID at baseline and after 28-days of l-arginine plus vitamin C or placebo supplementation enrolled in a randomized clinical trial, compared with a group of adults without previous history of SARS-CoV-2-infection. l-arginine-derived markers of nitric oxide (NO) bioavailability (i.e., l-arginine/ADMA, l-arginine/citrulline+ornithine, and l-arginine/ornithine) were also assayed. Partial least squares discriminant analysis (PLS-DA) models were built to characterize systemic l-arginine metabolism and assess the effects of the supplementation. PLS-DA allowed discrimination of participants with long COVID from healthy controls with 80.2 ± 3.0% accuracy. Lower markers of NO bioavailability were found in participants with long COVID. After 28 days of l-arginine plus vitamin C supplementation, serum l-arginine concentrations and l-arginine/ADMA increased significantly compared with placebo. This supplement may therefore be proposed as a remedy to increase NO bioavailability in people with long COVID.

https://pubmed.ncbi.nlm.nih.gov/36982151/

"L-arginine dysfunction is being seen in COVID patients and is associated with immune and vascular dysfunction."

Steven Magee

L-Citrulline

A Google search of 'pubmed 2023 long covid citrulline' produced no relevant findings. It appears there is little research being done in this area.

"COVID-19 is known to cause decreased levels of plasma citrulline."

Steven Magee

L-Lysine

A Google search of 'pubmed 2023 long covid lysine' produced no relevant findings. It appears there is little research being done in this area.

"Lysine is showing potential in treating COVID-19."

Steven Magee

Creatine

Reduced tissue creatine levels in patients with long COVID-19: A cross-sectional study...Total creatine concentration in the skeletal muscle and brain of long COVID patients were significantly lower when compared to the reference values for the general population, as measured with proton magnetic resonance spectroscopy at 1.5-T in vastus medialis muscle, thalamus, and three bilateral cerebral locations across the white and gray matter.

https://pubmed.ncbi.nlm.nih.gov/37171415/

Can creatine help in pulmonary rehabilitation after COVID-19?...COVID-19 pneumonia patients who responded successfully to intensive care treatments and were able to be discharged from hospital appear to experience a prolonged recovery, demanding resolute inpatient and outpatient rehabilitation services. Those include predominantly physiotherapy, occupational therapy, and speech-language retraining, with respect to recovery of the respiratory system as well as mobility and function. The recent European Society for Clinical Nutrition and Metabolism (ESPEN) concise guidance on clinical nutrition in COVID-19 patients properly addressed nutritional intervention and therapy as an integral part of the approach to patients victim to SARS-CoV-2 infection in the ICU setting, in an internal medicine ward setting as well as in general healthcare but omitted to consider nutritional guidance for COVID-19 survivors. Besides other early and short-term rehabilitative interventions, the International Task Force of the European Respiratory Society recently itemized adequate nutrition among rehabilitation needs for COVID-19 survivors upon release from hospital. Among other candidates, dietary creatine might emerge as one of the key elements of nutritional support following COVID-19 respiratory distress due to its beneficial effects demonstrated during rehabilitation in various lung conditions. For instance, creatine supplementation augments functional recovery during pulmonary rehabilitation in patients with chronic obstructive pulmonary disease, but also ameliorates cystic fibrosis, stroke, and respiratory failure, acting as an anti-inflammatory and energy-boosting agent. Although no disease-specific guidelines exist at present, a conventional creatine dosage of 5 g per day administered over 4 weeks or more might be risk-free and sufficient to back up pulmonary rehabilitation in COVID. Creatine is inexpensive, widely available, and has a favorable safety profile, therefore being a suitable promising compound that could meet a growing need for nutritional help during pulmonary rehabilitation in post-COVID-19 world.

https://www.ncbi.nlm.nih.gov/pmc/articles/PMC7649915/

Diagnostic and Pharmacological Potency of Creatine in Post-Viral Fatigue Syndrome...Post-viral fatigue syndrome (PVFS) is a widespread chronic neurological disease with no definite etiological factor(s), no actual diagnostic test, and no approved pharmacological treatment, therapy, or cure. Among other features, PVFS could be accompanied by various irregularities in creatine metabolism, perturbing either tissue levels of creatine in the brain, the rates of phosphocreatine resynthesis in the skeletal muscle, or the concentrations of the enzyme creatine kinase in the blood. Furthermore, supplemental creatine and related guanidino compounds appear to impact both patient- and clinician-reported outcomes in syndromes and maladies with chronic fatigue. This paper critically overviews the most common disturbances in creatine metabolism in various PVFS populations, summarizes human trials on dietary creatine and creatine analogs in the syndrome, and discusses new frontiers and open questions for using creatine in a post-COVID-19 world.

https://pubmed.ncbi.nlm.nih.gov/33557013/

Role of Creatine Supplementation in Conditions Involving Mitochondrial Dysfunction: A Narrative Review...Creatine monohydrate (CrM) is one of the most widely used nutritional supplements among active individuals and athletes to improve high-intensity exercise performance and training adaptations. However, research suggests that CrM supplementation may also serve as a therapeutic tool in the management of some chronic and traumatic diseases. Creatine supplementation has been reported to improve high-energy phosphate availability as well as have antioxidative, neuroprotective, anti-lactatic, and calcium-homoeostatic effects. These characteristics may have a direct impact on mitochondrion's survival and health particularly during stressful conditions such as ischemia and injury. This narrative review discusses current scientific evidence for use or supplemental CrM as a therapeutic agent during conditions associated with mitochondrial dysfunction. Based on this analysis, it appears that CrM supplementation may have a role in improving cellular bioenergetics in several mitochondrial dysfunction-related diseases, ischemic conditions, and injury pathology and thereby could provide therapeutic benefit in the management of these conditions. However, larger clinical trials are needed to explore these potential therapeutic applications before definitive conclusions can be drawn.

https://www.ncbi.nlm.nih.gov/pmc/articles/PMC8838971/

"Creatine levels tend to be lower in Long COVID patients."

Steven Magee

Organ Damage

Multi-organ impairment and long COVID: a 1-year prospective, longitudinal cohort study...Objectives: To determine the prevalence of organ impairment in long COVID patients at 6 and 12 months after initial symptoms and to explore links to clinical presentation. Design: Prospective cohort study. Participants: Individuals. Methods: In individuals recovered from acute COVID-19, we assessed symptoms, health status, and multi-organ tissue characterisation and function. Setting: Two non-acute healthcare settings (Oxford and London). Physiological and biochemical investigations were performed at baseline on all individuals, and those with organ impairment were reassessed. Main outcome measures: Primary outcome was prevalence of single- and multi-organ impairment at 6 and 12 months post COVID-19. Results: A total of 536 individuals (mean age 45 years, 73% female, 89% white, 32% healthcare workers, 13% acute COVID-19 hospitalisation) completed baseline assessment (median: 6 months post COVID-19); 331 (62%) with organ impairment or incidental findings had follow-up, with reduced symptom burden from baseline (median number of symptoms 10 and 3, at 6 and 12 months, respectively). Extreme breathlessness (38% and 30%), cognitive dysfunction (48% and 38%) and poor health-related quality of life (EQ-5D-5L < 0.7; 57% and 45%) were common at 6 and 12 months, and associated with female gender, younger age and single-organ impairment. Single- and multi-organ impairment were present in 69% and 23% at baseline, persisting in 59% and 27% at follow-up, respectively. Conclusions: Organ impairment persisted in 59% of 331 individuals followed up at 1 year post COVID-19, with implications for symptoms, quality of life and longer-term health, signalling the need for prevention and integrated care of long COVID.

https://pubmed.ncbi.nlm.nih.gov/36787802/

Organ and cell-specific biomarkers of Long-COVID identified with targeted proteomics and machine learning... Background: Survivors of acute COVID-19 often suffer prolonged, diffuse symptoms post-infection, referred to as "Long-COVID". A lack of Long-COVID biomarkers and pathophysiological mechanisms limits effective diagnosis, treatment and disease surveillance. We performed targeted proteomics and machine learning analyses to identify novel blood biomarkers of Long-COVID. Methods: A case-control study comparing the expression of 2925 unique blood proteins in Long-COVID outpatients versus COVID-19 inpatients and healthy control subjects. Targeted proteomics was accomplished with proximity extension assays, and machine learning was used to identify the most important proteins for identifying Long-COVID patients. Organ system and cell type expression patterns were identified with Natural Language Processing (NLP) of the UniProt Knowledgebase. Results: Machine learning analysis identified 119 relevant proteins for differentiating Long-COVID outpatients (Bonferonni corrected $P < 0.01$). Protein combinations were narrowed down to two optimal models, with nine and five proteins each, and with both having excellent sensitivity and specificity for Long-COVID status (AUC = 1.00, F1 = 1.00). NLP expression analysis highlighted the diffuse organ system involvement in Long-COVID, as well as the involved cell types, including leukocytes and platelets, as key components associated with Long-COVID. Conclusions: Proteomic analysis of plasma from Long-COVID patients identified 119 highly relevant proteins and two optimal models with nine and five proteins, respectively. The identified proteins reflected widespread organ and cell type expression. Optimal protein models, as well as individual proteins, hold the potential for accurate diagnosis of Long-COVID and targeted therapeutics.

https://pubmed.ncbi.nlm.nih.gov/36809921/

Post-COVID-19-associated multiorgan complications or "long COVID" with literature review and management strategy discussion: A meta-analysis... Objective: To investigate the post-COVID-19 long-term complications or long COVID of various organ systems in patients after 3 months of the infection, specifically before the Omicron variant, with comparative literature analysis. Methods: A systemic literature search and meta-analysis were conducted using multiple electronic databases (PubMed, Scopus, Cochrane library) with predefined search terms to identify eligible articles. Eligible studies reported long-term complications of COVID-19 infection before the Omicron variant infection. Case reports, case series, observational studies with cross-sectional or prospective research design, case-control studies, and experimental studies that reported post-COVID-19 complications were included. The complications reported after 3 months after the recovery from COVID-19 infection were included in the study. Results: The total number of studies available for analysis was 34. The effect size (ES) for neurological complications was 29% with 95% confidence interval (CI): 19%-39%. ES for psychiatric complications was 24% with 95% CI: 7%-41%. ES was 9% for cardiac outcomes, with a 95% CI of 1%-18%. ES was 22%, 95% CI: 5%-39% for the gastrointestinal outcome. ES for musculoskeletal symptoms was 18% with 95% CI: 9%-28%. ES for pulmonary complications was 28% with 95% CI: 18%-37%. ES for dermatological complications was 25%, with a 95% CI of 23%-26%. ES for endocrine outcomes was 8%, with a 95% CI of 8%-9%. ES size for renal outcomes was 3% with a 95% CI of 1%-7%. At the same time, other miscellaneous uncategorized outcomes had ES of 39% with 95% CI of 21%-57%. Apart from analyzing COVID-19 systemic complications outcomes, the ES for hospitalization and intensive care unit admissions were found to be 4%, 95% CI: 0%-7%, and 11% with 95% CI: 8%-14%. Conclusion: By acquiring the data and statistically analyzing the post-COVID-19 complications during the prevalence of most virulent strains, this study has generated a different way of understanding COVID-19 and its complications for better community health.

https://pubmed.ncbi.nlm.nih.gov/37064319/

Long COVID could become a widespread post-pandemic disease? A debate on the organs most

affected...Long COVID is an emerging problem in the current health care scenario. It is a syndrome with common symptoms of shortness of breath, fatigue, cognitive dysfunction, and other conditions that have a high impact on daily life. They are fluctuating or relapsing states that occur in patients with a history of SARS-CoV-2 infection for at least 2 months. They are usually conditions that at 3 months after onset cannot be explained by an alternative diagnosis. Currently very little is known about this syndrome. A thorough review of the literature highlights that the cause is attributable to deposits of tau protein. Massive phosphorylation of tau protein in response to SARS-CoV-2 infection occurred in brain samples from autopsies of people previously affected with COVID-19. The neurological disorders resulting from this clinical condition are termed tauopathies and can give different pathological symptoms depending on the involved anatomical region of the brain. Peripheral small-fiber neuropathies are also evident among patients with Long COVID leading to fatigue, which is the main symptom of this syndrome. Certainly more research studies could confirm the association between tau protein and Long COVID by defining the main role of tau protein as a biomarker for the diagnosis of this syndrome that is widespread in the post-pandemic period.

https://pubmed.ncbi.nlm.nih.gov/36773054/

"Organ damage is a common finding in Long COVID patients."

Steven Magee

Enzymes

A Randomized Controlled Trial of the Efficacy of Systemic Enzymes and Probiotics in the Resolution of Post-COVID Fatigue...Muscle fatigue and cognitive disturbances persist in patients after recovery from acute COVID-19 disease. However, there are no specific treatments for post-COVID fatigue. Objective: To evaluate the efficacy and safety of the health supplements ImmunoSEB (systemic enzyme complex) and ProbioSEB CSC3 (probiotic complex) in patients suffering from COVID-19 induced fatigue. A randomized, multicentric, double blind, placebo-controlled trial was conducted in 200 patients with a complaint of post-COVID fatigue. The test arm (n = 100) received the oral supplements for 14 days and the control arm (n = 100) received a placebo. Treatment efficacy was compared using the Chalder Fatigue scale (CFQ-11), at various time points from days 1 to 14. The supplemental treatment resulted in resolution of fatigue in a greater percentage of subjects in the test vs. the control arm (91% vs. 15%) on day 14. Subjects in the test arm showed a significantly greater reduction in total as well as physical and mental fatigue scores at all time points vs. the control arm. The supplements were well tolerated with no adverse events reported. This study demonstrates that a 14 days supplementation of ImmunoSEB + ProbioSEB CSC3 resolves post-COVID-19 fatigue and can improve patients' functional status and quality of life.

https://www.ncbi.nlm.nih.gov/pmc/articles/PMC8472462/

Notes:

- ImmunoSEB™ is a blend of Peptizyme SP™ (serrapeptase), Bromelain, Amylase, Lysozyme, Peptidase, Glucoamylase, Catalase, Papain, Lactoferrin.

    - https://immunoseb.com/what-is-immunoseb/

- ProbioSEB CSC3™. Triple strength blend with SEBtilis™ (Bacillus subtilis), SEBiotic™ (Bacillus coagulans), and SEBclausii™ (Bacillus clausii), gram-positive bacteria that supports healthy immune function.
  - https://specialtyenzymes.com/products/probiotics/probioseb-csc3/

The enzymes in COVID-19: A review...As enzymes are indispensable to uncountable biochemical reactions in the human body, it is not surprising that some enzymes are of relevance to COVID-19 pathophysiology. Past evidence from SARS-CoV and MERS-CoV outbreaks provided hints about the role of enzymes in SARS-CoV-2 infection. In this setting, ACE-2 is an enzyme of great importance since it is the cell entry receptor for SARS-CoV-2. Clinical data elucidate patterns of enzymatic alterations in COVID-19, which could be associated with organ damage, prognosis, and clinical complications. Further, viral mutations can create new disease behaviors, and these effects are related to the activity of enzymes. This review will discuss the main enzymes related to COVID-19, summarizing the findings on their role in viral entry mechanism, the consequences of their dysregulation, and the effects of SARS-CoV-2 mutations on them.

https://www.ncbi.nlm.nih.gov/pmc/articles/PMC8789385/

The Pathophysiology of Long COVID throughout the Renin-Angiotensin System...Long COVID is a term coined by the World Health Organization (WHO) to describe a variety of persistent symptoms after acute SARS-CoV-2 infection. Long COVID has been demonstrated to affect various SARS-CoV-2-infected persons, independently of the acute disease severity. The symptoms of long COVID, like acute COVID-19, consist in the set of damage to various organs and systems such as the respiratory, cardiovascular, neurological, endocrine, urinary, and immune systems. Fatigue, dyspnea, cardiac abnormalities, cognitive and attention impairments, sleep disturbances, post-traumatic stress disorder, muscle pain, concentration problems, and headache were all reported as symptoms of long COVID. At the molecular level, the renin-angiotensin system (RAS) is heavily involved in the pathogenesis of this illness, much as it is in the acute phase of the viral infection. In this review, we summarize the impact of long COVID on several organs and tissues, with a special focus on the significance of the RAS in the disease pathogenesis. Long COVID risk factors and potential therapy approaches are also explored.

https://pubmed.ncbi.nlm.nih.gov/35566253/

"Dysregulation of enzymes is known to occur in COVID infections."

Steven Magee

Digestive System

Digestive involvement in the Long-COVID syndrome…The SARS-CoV-2 infection which caused a worldwide epidemic was considered first a lung disease. Later on, it was found that the disease caused by this virus, SARS-CoV-2, can affect most organs, including the digestive system. The long-term effects of this infection are now progressively detected and called Long-COVID. This review aims is to present the updated knowledge of the digestive sequelae after SARS-CoV-2 infection…The main symptoms that can occur in the long term are: diarrhea, nausea, vomiting, abdominal pain, along with increased liver enzymes. Patients with chronic diseases have a higher risk of developing long-term sequelae, but it is not documented that digestive sequelae are influenced by the presence of chronic diseases.

https://www.ncbi.nlm.nih.gov/pmc/articles/PMC9177081/

Long-term gastrointestinal outcomes of COVID-19…A comprehensive evaluation of the risks and 1-year burdens of gastrointestinal disorders in the post-acute phase of COVID-19 is needed but is not yet available. Here we use the US Department of Veterans Affairs national health care databases to build a cohort of 154,068 people with COVID-19, 5,638,795 contemporary controls, and 5,859,621 historical controls to estimate the risks and 1-year burdens of a set of pre-specified incident gastrointestinal outcomes. We show that beyond the first 30 days of infection, people with COVID-19 exhibited increased risks and 1-year burdens of incident gastrointestinal disorders spanning several disease categories including motility disorders, acid related disorders (dyspepsia, gastroesophageal reflux disease, peptic ulcer disease), functional intestinal disorders, acute pancreatitis, hepatic and biliary disease. The risks were evident in people who were not hospitalized during the acute phase of COVID-19 and increased in a graded fashion across the severity spectrum of the acute phase of COVID-

19 (non-hospitalized, hospitalized, and admitted to intensive care). The risks were consistent in comparisons including the COVID-19 vs the contemporary control group and COVID-19 vs the historical control group as the referent category. Altogether, our results show that people with SARS-CoV-2 infection are at increased risk of gastrointestinal disorders in the post-acute phase of COVID-19. Post-covid care should involve attention to gastrointestinal health and disease.

https://pubmed.ncbi.nlm.nih.gov/36882400/

Long-term Gastrointestinal Sequelae Following COVID-19: A Prospective Follow-up Cohort

Study...Background & aims: Coronavirus disease 2019 (COVID-19) is associated with long-term gastrointestinal sequelae; however, prospective longitudinal data are sparse. We prospectively studied the frequency, spectrum, and risk factors of post infection functional gastrointestinal disorders/disorders of gut-brain interaction (PI-FGID/DGBI) after COVID-19. Methods: Three hundred twenty cases with COVID-19 and 2 control groups, group A, 320 healthy spouses/family controls, and group B, 280 healthy COVID serology-negative controls, were prospectively followed up at 1, 3, and 6 months by using validated Rome IV criteria to evaluate the frequency of PI-FGID/DGBI. Results: Of 320 cases, at 1 month 36 (11.3%) developed FGID symptoms. Persistent symptoms were noted in 27 (8.4%) at 3 months and in 21 (6.6%) at 6 months. At 3 months, 8 (2.5%) had irritable bowel syndrome, 7 (2.2%) had functional diarrhea, 6 (1.9%) had functional dyspepsia, 3 (0.9%) had functional constipation, 2 (0.6%) had functional dyspepsia-IBS overlap, and 1 (0.3%) had functional abdominal bloating/distention. Among symptomatic individuals at 3 months, 8 (29.6%) were positive for isolated carbohydrate malabsorption, 1 (3.7%) was positive for post infection malabsorption syndrome, and 1 (3.7%) was positive for intestinal methanogen overgrowth. None of the healthy controls developed FGID up to 6 months of follow-up (P < .01). Predictive factors at 3 and 6 months were severity of infection (P < .01) and presence of gastrointestinal symptoms at the time of infection (P < .01). Conclusions:

COVID-19 led to significantly higher number of new onset PI-FGID/DGBI compared with healthy controls at 3 and 6 months of follow-up. If further investigated, some patients can be diagnosed with underlying malabsorption.

https://pubmed.ncbi.nlm.nih.gov/36273799/

Post-COVID-19 Gastro-Intestinal Disturbances

...Background: Since the end of 2019, SARS-CoV-2 has been responsible for the multisystemic hyper-inflammatory disease, namely, COVID-19, as a majorly impactful pandemic. Gastrointestinal (GI) symptoms occurring during and after disease are gaining increasing attention among experts. Methods: We briefly review and comment on preliminary and recent evidences on prevalence, pathophysiology, and perspective treatment options for GI disturbances during and after COVID-19. Results: Several reports from the literature show a significant portion of COVID-19 patients suffering from GI symptoms both at the early stages of the disease and after the end of it, sometimes for several months, namely "long-COVID-19" patients, irrespective of vaccination. An unsolved issue regarding COVID-19 is the association between GI symptoms and the outcome of COVID-19 patients. Several studies and metanalyses suggest a worse evolution of COVID-19 in patients presenting with GI symptoms. However, these data have not been agreed. Indeed, only one uniform observation can be found in the literature: patients with chronic liver disease have a worse outcome from COVID-19 infection. Upper and lower GI symptoms have similarities with postinfectious functional dyspepsia (FD) and irritable bowel syndrome (IBS). FD and IBS following infection are recognize as pathophysiological factor the gut microbial, which is a gut microbial quali- and quantitative unbalance, namely dysbiosis. Furthermore, several preliminary reports and ongoing clinical trials have shown gut microbiota modulation by pre-, pro- and postbiotics to be effective in changing and preventing COVID-19 natural course. Conclusion: GI symptoms characterize both long- and non-long-COVID-19 with a potentially significant impact on its natural course. Gut microbiota modulation seems to be a sensible target for disease treatment and/or prevention.

https://pubmed.ncbi.nlm.nih.gov/36464877/

Gastrointestinal manifestations of long COVID: A systematic review and meta-analysis...Background: Prolonged symptoms after COVID-19 are an important concern due to the large numbers affected by the pandemic. Objectives: To ascertain the frequency of gastrointestinal (GI) manifestations as part of long GI COVID. Design: A systematic review and meta-analysis of studies reporting GI manifestations in long COVID was performed. Data sources and methods: Electronic databases (Medline, Scopus, Embase, Cochrane Central Register of Controlled Trials, and Web of Science) were searched till 21 December 2021 to identify studies reporting frequency of GI symptoms in long COVID. We included studies reporting overall GI manifestations or individual GI symptoms as part of long COVID. We excluded pediatric studies and those not providing relevant information. We calculated the pooled frequency of various symptoms in all patients with COVID-19 and also in those with long COVID using the inverse variance approach. All analysis was done using R version 4.1.1 using packages 'meta' and 'metafor'. Results: A total of 50 studies were included. The frequencies of GI symptoms were 0.12 [95% confidence interval (CI), 0.06-0.22, I 2 = 99%] and 0.22 (95% CI, 0.10-0.41, I 2 = 97%) in patients with COVID-19 and those with long COVID, respectively. The frequencies of abdominal pain, nausea/vomiting, loss of appetite, and loss of taste were 0.14 (95% CI, 0.04-0.38, I 2 = 96%), 0.06 (95% CI, 0.03-0.11, I 2 = 98%), 0.20 (95% CI, 0.08-0.43, I 2 = 98%), and 0.17 (95% CI, 0.10-0.27, I 2 = 95%), respectively, after COVID-19. The frequencies of diarrhea, dyspepsia, and irritable bowel syndrome were 0.10 (95% CI, 0.04-0.23, I 2 = 98%), 0.20 (95% CI, 0.06-0.50, I 2 = 97%), and 0.17 (95% CI, 0.06-0.37, I 2 = 96%), respectively. Conclusion: GI symptoms in patients were seen in 12% after COVID-19 and 22% as part of long COVID. Loss of appetite, dyspepsia, irritable bowel syndrome, loss of taste, and abdominal pain were the five most common GI symptoms of long COVID.

https://pubmed.ncbi.nlm.nih.gov/36004306/

"Digestive issues are a feature of Long COVID."

Steven Magee

Kidneys

Long COVID: Is there a kidney link?...Metabolic causes such as altered bioenergetics and amino acid metabolism may play a major role in Long COVID. Renal-metabolic regulation is an integral part of these pathways but has not been systematically or routinely investigated in Long COVID. Here we discuss the biochemistry of renal tubular injury as it may contribute to Long COVID symptoms. We propose three potential mechanisms that could be involved in Long COVID namely creatine phosphate metabolism, un-reclaimed glomerular filtrate and COVID specific proximal tubule cells (PTC) injury-a tryptophan paradigm. This approach is intended to allow for improved diagnostics and therapy for the long-haul sufferers.

https://pubmed.ncbi.nlm.nih.gov/37077670/

Kidney Outcomes in Long COVID...Patients who survive coronavirus disease 2019 (COVID-19) are at higher risk of post-acute sequelae involving pulmonary and several extrapulmonary organ systems—generally referred to as long COVID. However, a detailed assessment of kidney outcomes in long COVID is not yet available. Here we show that, beyond the acute phase of illness, 30-day survivors of COVID-19 exhibited higher risks of AKI, eGFR decline, ESKD, major adverse kidney events (MAKE), and steeper longitudinal decline in eGFR. The risks of kidney outcomes increased according to the severity of the acute infection (categorized by care setting into non-hospitalized, hospitalized, and admitted to intensive care). The findings provide insight into the long-term consequences of COVID-19 on kidney outcomes and suggest that post-acute COVID-19 care should include attention to kidney function and disease...The implications of our findings are clear. Given the large number of people infected with COVID-19 (>43 million people in the United States, and >234 million globally), and given that estimates by the World Health Organization suggest that around 10% of people infected with COVID-19 may experience post-acute sequelae, the numbers of people with long COVID-19 in need of post–COVID-19 care will likely be staggering and will present substantial strain on already overwhelmed health systems. Governments and health systems around the world are establishing post-acute COVID-19 clinics to attend to the needs of people with postacute COVID-19 sequelae. The optimal composition of those clinics is not yet clear. The higher risks of adverse kidney outcomes reported in this study highlights the need for integration of kidney care as a component of the multidisciplinary post-acute COVID-19 care. Our estimates of the burden of kidney sequelae may also be useful to inform capacity planning.

https://www.ncbi.nlm.nih.gov/pmc/articles/PMC8806085/

Long-term interplay between COVID-19 and chronic kidney disease...Purpose: The COVID-19 pandemic may have an impact on the long-term kidney function of survivors. The clinical relevance is not clear. Methods: This review summarises the currently published data. Results: There is a bidirectional relationship between chronic kidney disease and COVID-19 disease. Chronic kidney diseases due to primary kidney disease or chronic conditions affecting kidneys increase the susceptibility to COVID-19 infection, the risks for progression and critical COVID-19 disease (with acute or acute-on-chronic kidney damage), and death. Patients who have survived COVID-19 face an increased risk of worse kidney outcomes in the post-acute phase of the disease. Of clinical significance, COVID-19 may predispose surviving patients to chronic kidney disease, independently of clinically apparent acute kidney injury (AKI). The increased risk of post-acute renal dysfunction of COVID-19 patients can be graded according to the severity of the acute infection (non-hospitalised, hospitalised or ICU patients). The burden of chronic kidney disease developing after COVID-19 is currently unknown. Conclusion: Post-acute COVID-19 care should include close attention to kidney function. Future prospective large-scale studies are needed with long and complete follow-up periods, assessing kidney function using novel markers of kidney function/damage, urinalysis and biopsy studies.

https://pubmed.ncbi.nlm.nih.gov/36828919/

Long-term kidney function recovery and mortality after COVID-19-associated acute kidney injury: An international multi-centre observational cohort study...Background: While acute kidney injury (AKI) is a common complication in COVID-19, data on post-AKI kidney function recovery and the clinical factors associated with poor kidney function recovery is lacking. Methods: A retrospective multi-centre observational cohort study comprising 12,891 hospitalized patients aged 18 years or older with a diagnosis of SARS-CoV-2 infection confirmed by polymerase chain reaction from 1 January 2020 to 10 September 2020, and with at least one serum creatinine value 1-365 days prior to admission. Mortality and serum creatinine values were obtained up to 10 September 2021. Findings: Advanced age (HR 2.77, 95%CI 2.53-3.04, p < 0.0001), severe COVID-19 (HR 2.91, 95%CI 2.03-4.17, p < 0.0001), severe AKI (KDIGO stage 3: HR 4.22, 95%CI 3.55-5.00, p < 0.0001), and ischemic heart disease (HR 1.26, 95%CI 1.14-1.39, p < 0.0001) were associated with worse mortality outcomes. AKI severity (KDIGO stage 3: HR 0.41, 95%CI 0.37-0.46, p < 0.0001) was associated with worse kidney function recovery, whereas remdesivir use (HR 1.34, 95%CI 1.17-1.54, p < 0.0001) was associated with better kidney function recovery. In a subset of patients without chronic kidney disease, advanced age (HR 1.38, 95%CI 1.20-1.58, p < 0.0001), male sex (HR 1.67, 95%CI 1.45-1.93, p < 0.0001), severe AKI (KDIGO stage 3: HR 11.68, 95%CI 9.80-13.91, p < 0.0001), and hypertension (HR 1.22, 95%CI 1.10-1.36, p = 0.0002) were associated with post-AKI kidney function impairment. Furthermore, patients with COVID-19-associated AKI had significant and persistent elevations of baseline serum creatinine 125% or more at 180 days (RR 1.49, 95%CI 1.32-1.67) and 365 days (RR 1.54, 95%CI 1.21-1.96) compared to COVID-19 patients with no AKI. Interpretation: COVID-19-associated AKI was associated with higher mortality, and severe COVID-19-associated

AKI was associated with worse long-term post-AKI kidney function recovery.

https://pubmed.ncbi.nlm.nih.gov/36381999/

Long COVID and kidney disease...Kidney involvement is common in patients with acute SARS-CoV-2 infection, and subclinical inflammation and injury may persist for many months, resulting in a progressive decline in kidney function that leads to chronic kidney disease. Continued research is imperative to understand these long-term sequelae and identify interventions to mitigate them.

https://pubmed.ncbi.nlm.nih.gov/34504319/

"The kidneys are commonly damaged during coronavirus infections."

Steven Magee

Liver

Long COVID-19 Liver Manifestation in Children...OBJECTIVES: Severe acute respiratory syndrome coronavirus 2, the novel coronavirus responsible for coronavirus disease (COVID-19), has been a major cause of morbidity and mortality worldwide. Gastrointestinal and hepatic manifestations during acute disease have been reported extensively in the literature. Post-COVID-19 cholangiopathy has been increasingly reported in adults. In children, data are sparse. Our aim was to describe pediatric patients who recovered from COVID-19 and later presented with liver injury. METHODS: This is a retrospective case series study of pediatric patients with post-COVID-19 liver manifestations. We collected data on demographics, medical history, clinical presentation, laboratory results, imaging, histology, treatment, and outcome. RESULTS: We report 5 pediatric patients who recovered from COVID-19 and later presented with liver injury. Two types of clinical presentation were distinguishable. Two infants aged 3 and 5 months, previously healthy, presented with acute liver failure that rapidly progressed to liver transplantation. Their liver explant showed massive necrosis with cholangiolar proliferation and lymphocytic infiltrate. Three children, 2 aged 8 years and 1 aged 13 years, presented with hepatitis with cholestasis. Two children had a liver biopsy significant for lymphocytic portal and parenchyma inflammation, along with bile duct proliferations. All 3 were started on steroid treatment; liver enzymes improved, and they were weaned successfully from treatment. For all 5 patients, extensive etiology workup for infectious and metabolic etiologies was negative. CONCLUSIONS: We report 2 distinct patterns of potentially long COVID-19 liver manifestations in children with common clinical, radiological, and histopathological characteristics after a thorough workup excluded other known etiologies.

https://www.ncbi.nlm.nih.gov/research/coronavirus/publication/35687535

Long-term clinical outcomes of patients with COVID-19 and chronic liver disease: US multicenter COLD study

...Background: COVID-19 is associated with higher morbidity and mortality in patients with chronic liver diseases (CLDs). However, our understanding of the long-term outcomes of COVID-19 in patients with CLD is limited. Methods: We conducted a multicenter, observational cohort study of adult patients with CLD who were diagnosed with COVID-19 before May 30, 2020, to determine long-term clinical outcomes. We used a control group of patients with CLD confirmed negative for COVID-19. Results: We followed 666 patients with CLD (median age 58 years, 52.8% male) for a median of 384 (interquartile range: 31-462) days. The long-term mortality was 8.1%; with 3.6% experiencing delayed COVID-19-related mortality. Compared to a propensity-matched control group of patients with CLD without COVID-19 (n=1332), patients with CLD with COVID-19 had worse long-term survival [p<0.001; hazards ratio (HR): 1.69; 95% CI: 1.19-2.41] and higher rate of hospitalization (p<0.001, HR: 2.00, 1.62-2.48) over a 1-year follow-up period. Overall, 29.9% of patients reported symptoms of long-COVID-19. On multivariable analysis, female sex (p=0.05, HR: 2.45, 1.01-2.11), Hispanic ethnicity (p=0.003, HR: 1.94, 1.26-2.99), and severe COVID-19 requiring mechanical ventilation (p=0.028, HR: 1.74, 1.06-2.86) predicted long-COVID-19. In survivors, liver-related laboratory parameters showed significant improvement after COVID-19 resolution. COVID-19 vaccine status was available for 72% (n=470) of patients with CLD and history of COVID-19, of whom, 70% (n=326) had received the COVID-19 vaccine. Conclusions: Our large, longitudinal, multicenter study demonstrates a high burden of long-term mortality and morbidity in patients with CLD and COVID-19. Symptoms consistent with long-COVID-19 were present in 30% of patients with CLD. These results illustrate the prolonged implications of COVID-19 both for recovering patients and for health care systems.

https://pubmed.ncbi.nlm.nih.gov/36633476/

Liver Function in Patients with Long-Term Coronavirus Disease 2019 of up to 20 Months: A Cross-Sectional Study...The long-term laboratory aspects of the effects of coronavirus disease 2019 (COVID-19) on liver function are still not well understood. Therefore, this study aimed to evaluate the hepatic clinical laboratory profile of patients with up to 20 months of long-term COVID-19. A total of 243 patients of both sexes aged 18 years or older admitted during the acute phase of COVID-19 were included in this study. Liver function analysis was performed. Changes were identified in the mean levels of alanine aminotransferase (ALT), aspartate aminotransferase (AST), lactate dehydrogenase (LDH), gamma-glutamyl transferase (GGT), and ferritin. A ferritin level of >300 U/L was observed in the group that presented more changes in liver function markers (ALT, AST, and GGT). Age ≥ 60 years, male sex, AST level > 25 U/L, and GGT level ≥ 50 or 32 U/L were associated with an ALT level > 29 U/L. A correlation was found between ALT and AST, LDH, GGT, and ferritin. Our findings suggest that ALT and AST levels may be elevated in patients with long-term COVID-19, especially in those hospitalised during the acute phase. In addition, an ALT level > 29 U/L was associated with changes in the levels of other markers of liver injury, such as LDH, GGT, and ferritin.

https://pubmed.ncbi.nlm.nih.gov/37047897/

COVID-19 and liver injury: An ongoing challenge...Although COVID-19 is presented, usually, with typical respiratory symptoms (i.e., dyspnea, cough) and fever, extrapulmonary manifestations are also encountered. Liver injury is a common feature in patients with COVID-19 and ranges from mild and temporary elevation of liver enzymes to severe liver injury and, even, acute liver failure. The pathogenesis of liver damage is not clearly defined; multiple mechanisms contribute to liver disorder, including direct cytopathic viral effect, cytokine storm and immune-mediated hepatitis, hypoxic injury, and drug-induced liver toxicity. Patients with underlying chronic liver disease (i.e., cirrhosis, non-alcoholic fatty liver disease, alcohol-related liver disease, hepatocellular carcinoma, etc.) may have greater risk to develop both severe COVID-19 and further liver deterioration, and, as a consequence, certain issues should be considered during disease management. The aim of this review is to present the prevalence, clinical manifestation and pathophysiological mechanisms of liver injury in patients with SARS-CoV-2 infection. Moreover, we overview the association between chronic liver disease and SARS-CoV-2 infection and we briefly discuss the management of liver injury during COVID-19.

https://pubmed.ncbi.nlm.nih.gov/36687117/

"Liver damage was common in Long COVID."

Steven Magee

Damaged Liver Or Kidneys?

So you have long COVID and are wondering if you have liver and/or kidney damage? How do you know which damage you may have? The damaged liver may produce the following symptoms:

- Cognitive dysfunction:
  - Encephalopathy.
  - Unusual changes in mental state.
  - Personality changes.
  - Behavioral issues.
  - Confusion.
  - Disorientation.
  - Changes in mood.
  - Mood swings.
  - Irritability.
  - Headaches.
  - Ataxia.
  - Poor concentration.
  - Memory problems.
  - Flapping hands.
  - Handwriting issues.
  - Difficulty with mathematics.
  - Crankiness.
  - Tremors.
  - Seizures.
  - Coma.

- Sleep:
  - Sleeping issues.
  - Sleepiness.
  - Excessive sleepiness.
- Gastrointestinal:
  - Breath may have a musty or sweet odor.
  - Gas in the intestinal tract.
  - Feel sick to your stomach.
  - Nausea.
  - Vomiting.
  - Vomiting blood.
  - Loss of appetite.
  - Pale stool color.
  - Abdominal pain and swelling.
  - Ascites.
  - Esophageal bleeding varices.
  - Weight loss.
  - Tenderness in the upper abdomen.
- Skin:
  - Jaundice.
  - Edema.
  - Itchy skin.
  - Bruise easily.
  - Blood vessels visible in the skin.
- Blood:
  - Abnormal bleeding.
  - Easy bleeding.

- ○ Coagulopathy.
- A general unwell feeling.
- Hyperammonemia.
- Hyperventilation.
- Dark urine color.
- Fluid retention.
- Chronic fatigue.
- Feeling tired.
- Feeling weak.
- Muscle weakness.
- Loss of sex drive.
- Portal hypertension.
- Liver enlargement.
- Cholestasis.
- Chills.
- Babies:
  - ○ Irritability.
  - ○ Vomiting.
  - ○ Lethargy.
  - ○ Seizures.
  - ○ Grunting when breathing.
  - ○ Hyperventilation.
- Children:
  - ○ Failure to thrive.
  - ○ Hypotonia.
  - ○ Neurodevelopmental delays.

The damaged kidneys may produce the following symptoms of uremia:

- Cognitive dysfunction:
    - Trouble concentrating.
    - Abnormal behavior.
    - Confusion.
    - Disorientation.
    - Headache.
    - Depression.
    - Stroke.
    - Uremic encephalopathy.
- Fatigue:
    - Extreme fatigue.
    - Extreme tiredness.
    - Drowsiness.
- Heart:
    - Chest pain.
    - Angina.
    - Atherosclerosis.
    - Heart failure.
    - Heart valve disease.
    - Pericardial effusion.
    - High blood pressure.
    - Heart disease.
    - Death by heart attack.
- Lungs:

- ○ Shortness of breath from fluid accumulation.
- ○ Pulmonary edema.
- ○ Difficulty breathing.
- Blood:
  - ○ Defective platelet function.
  - ○ Blood clotting leading to bleeding.
  - ○ Anemia.
- Gastrointestinal:
  - ○ Loss of appetite.
  - ○ Nausea
  - ○ Vomiting.
  - ○ Unexplained weight loss.
  - ○ Malnutrition.
- Kidneys:
  - ○ Uremic fetor (a urine-like odor on the breath or metallic taste in the mouth).
  - ○ Uremic frost (yellow-white crystals on the skin due to urea in sweat).
  - ○ Kidney stones.
  - ○ Kidney disease.
- Muscle cramps.
- Itching.
- Acidosis.
- Hyperkalemia.
- Hyperparathyroidism.
- Hypothyroidism.
- Infertility.

- Gout.

- Diabetes.

- Metabolic syndrome.

- Amyloidosis.

Damage to the liver and/or kidneys may cause urea cycle disorders. A damaged liver will produce hyperammonemia and damaged kidneys will produce uremia in the body. You are being poisoned by your own body! It is important to identify and correctly treat organ damage prior to it progressing into severe disabling illness that may lead to premature death.

"Organ damage is a common outcome of a coronavirus infection and should be suspected in people that are not recovering their health afterwards."

Steven Magee

Food Intolerance & Allergies

Long COVID: pathophysiological factors and abnormalities of coagulation...Acute COVID-19 infection is followed by prolonged symptoms in approximately one in ten cases: known as Long COVID. The disease affects ~65 million individuals worldwide. Many pathophysiological processes appear to underlie Long COVID, including viral factors (persistence, reactivation, and bacteriophagic action of SARS CoV-2); host factors (chronic inflammation, metabolic and endocrine dysregulation, immune dysregulation, and autoimmunity); and downstream impacts (tissue damage from the initial infection, tissue hypoxia, host dysbiosis, and autonomic nervous system dysfunction). These mechanisms culminate in the long-term persistence of the disorder characterized by a thrombotic endothelialitis, endothelial inflammation, hyperactivated platelets, and fibrinaloid microclots. These abnormalities of blood vessels and coagulation affect every organ system and represent a unifying pathway for the various symptoms of Long COVID....Mast cell activation. The hyperinflammatory responses in acute COVID-19 infection and Long COVID have been hypothesized to be facilitated, in part, by mast cell activation. Mast cell activation can escalate into mast cell activation syndrome (MCAS), which causes repeated severe allergic symptoms affecting several body systems. Unregulated release of chemical mediators produces a multitude of symptoms, including food allergies, urticaria, gastrointestinal upset, shortness of breath, and wheezing, all of which are reported in Long COVID. The proposed mechanisms whereby MCAS is triggered in Long COVID include dysregulation of genes by SARS-CoV-2, resulting in the loss of genetic regulation of mast cells, as well as development of autoantibodies which react with immunoglobulin receptors on mast cells.

https://www.ncbi.nlm.nih.gov/pmc/articles/PMC10113134/

Mast cell activation syndrome and the link with long COVID...Mast cells are innate immune cells found in connective tissues throughout the body, most prevalent at tissue-environment interfaces. They possess multiple cell-surface receptors which react to various stimuli and, after activation, release many mediators including histamine, heparin, cytokines, prostaglandins, leukotrienes and proteases. In mast cell activation syndrome, excessive amounts of inflammatory mediators are released in response to triggers such as foods, fragrances, stress, exercise, medications or temperature changes. Diagnostic markers may be difficult to assess because of their rapid degradation; these include urinary N-methyl histamine, urinary prostaglandins D2, DM and F2α and serum tryptase (which is stable) in the UK. Self-management techniques, medications and avoiding triggers may improve quality of life. Treatments include mast cell mediator blockers, mast cell stabilisers and anti-inflammatory agents. 'Long COVID' describes post-COVID-19 syndrome when symptoms persist for more than 12 weeks after initial infection with no alternative diagnosis. Both mast cell activation syndrome and long COVID cause multiple symptoms. It is theorised that COVID-19 infection could lead to exaggeration of existing undiagnosed mast cell activation syndrome, or could activate normal mast cells owing to the persistence of viral particles. Other similarities include the relapse-remission cycle and improvements with similar treatments. Importantly, however, aside from mast cell disorders, long COVID could potentially be attributed to several other conditions.

https://pubmed.ncbi.nlm.nih.gov/35938771/

Mast cell activation symptoms are prevalent in Long-COVID...Hyper-inflammation caused by COVID-19 may be mediated by mast cell activation (MCA) which has also been hypothesized to cause Long-COVID (LC) symptoms...MCA symptoms were increased in LC and mimicked the symptoms and severity reported by patients who have mast cell activation syndrome (MCAS). Increased activation of aberrant mast cells induced by SARS-CoV-2 infection by various mechanisms may underlie part of the pathophysiology of LC, possibly suggesting routes to effective therapy.

https://pubmed.ncbi.nlm.nih.gov/34563706/

"Progressing food intolerance that would trigger fatigue and sleepiness was a big feature of my Long COVID symptoms."

Steven Magee

Fungal Infections

Long COVID: major findings, mechanisms and recommendations...Higher levels of fungal translocation, from the gut and/or lung epithelium, have been found in the plasma of patients with long COVID compared with those without long COVID or SARS-CoV-2-negative controls, possibly inducing cytokine production. Transferring gut bacteria from patients with long COVID to healthy mice resulted in lost cognitive functioning and impaired lung defences in the mice, who were partially treated with the commensal probiotic bacterium Bifidobacterium longum.

https://www.ncbi.nlm.nih.gov/pmc/articles/PMC9839201/

Endogenous Fungal Endophthalmitis following COVID-19 Hospitalization: Evidence from a Year-Long Observational Study...Purpose: To describe cases of endogenous fungal endophthalmitis (EFE) post-recovery from or hospitalization for coronavirus disease 2019 (COVID-19). Methods: This prospective audit involved patients with suspected endophthalmitis referred to a tertiary eye care center over a one-year period. Comprehensive ocular examinations, laboratory studies, and imaging were performed. Confirmed cases of EFE with a recent history of COVID-19 hospitalization±intensive care unit admission were identified, documented, managed, followed up, and described. Results: Seven eyes of six patients were reported; 5/6 were male, and the mean age was 55. The mean duration of hospitalization for COVID-19 was approximately 28 days (14-45); the mean time from discharge to onset of visual symptoms was 22 days (0-35). All patients had underlying conditions (5/6 hypertension; 3/6 diabetes mellitus; 2/6 asthma) and had received dexamethasone and remdesivir during their COVID-related hospitalization. All presented with decreased vision, and 4/6 complained of floaters. Baseline visual acuity ranged from light perception (LP) to counting fingers (CF). The fundus was not visible in 3 out of 7 eyes; the other 4 had "creamy-white fluffy lesions" at the posterior pole as well as significant vitritis. Vitreous taps were positive for Candida species in six and Aspergillus species in one eye. Anti-fungal treatment included intravenous amphotericin B followed by oral voriconazole and intravitreal amphotericin B. Three eyes underwent vitrectomy; the systemic health of two patients precluded surgery. One patient (with aspergillosis) died; the others were followed for 7-10 months - the final visual outcome improved from CF to 20/200-20/50 in 4 eyes and worsened (hand motion to LP) or did not change (LP), in two others. Conclusion: Ophthalmologists should maintain a high index of clinical suspicion for EFE in cases with visual symptoms and a history of recent COVID-19 hospitalization and/or systemic corticosteroid use - even without other well-known risk factors.

https://pubmed.ncbi.nlm.nih.gov/36890074/

Characterization of oral bacterial and fungal microbiome in recovered COVID-19 patients...COVID-19 has emerged as a global pandemic, challenging the world's economic and health systems. Human oral microbiota comprises the second largest microbial community after the gut microbiota and is closely related to respiratory tract infections; however, oral microbiomes of patients who have recovered from COVID-19 have not yet been thoroughly studied. Herein, we compared the oral bacterial and fungal microbiota after clearance of SARS-CoV-2 in 23 COVID-19 recovered patients to those of 29 healthy individuals. Our results showed that both bacterial and fungal diversity were nearly normalized in recovered patients. The relative abundance of some specific bacteria and fungi, primarily opportunistic pathogens, decreased in recovered patients (RPs), while the abundance of butyrate-producing organisms increased in these patients. Moreover, these differences were still present for some organisms at 12 months after recovery, indicating the need for long-term monitoring of COVID-19 patients after virus clearance.

https://pubmed.ncbi.nlm.nih.gov/37158877/

"Fungal infections were being seen during COVID-19."

Steven Magee

Monster Energy Drink

Green "Monster Energy" drink contains the following:
- Riboflavin (B2) 260%.
- Niacin (B3) 250%.
- Vitamin B6 240%.
- Vitamin B12 500%.
- Glucose.
- Taurine.
- Panax ginger extract.
- L-Carnitine.
- Caffeine.
- Glucuronolactone.
- Inositol.
- Gurana extract.
- Maltodextrin.

A multi-omics based anti-inflammatory immune signature characterizes long COVID-19 syndrome...To investigate long COVID-19 syndrome (LCS) pathophysiology, we performed an exploratory study with blood plasma derived from three groups: 1) healthy vaccinated individuals without SARS-CoV-2 exposure; 2) asymptomatic recovered patients at least three months after SARS-CoV-2 infection and; 3) symptomatic patients at least 3 months after SARS-CoV-2 infection with chronic fatigue syndrome or similar symptoms, here designated as patients with long COVID-19 syndrome (LCS). Multiplex cytokine profiling indicated slightly elevated pro-inflammatory cytokine levels in recovered individuals in contrast to patients with LCS. Plasma proteomics demonstrated low levels of acute phase proteins and macrophage-derived secreted proteins in LCS. High levels of anti-inflammatory oxylipins including omega-3 fatty acids in LCS were detected by eicosadomics, whereas targeted metabolic profiling indicated high levels of anti-inflammatory osmolytes taurine and hypaphorine, but low amino acid and triglyceride levels and deregulated acylcarnitines. A model considering alternatively polarized macrophages as a major contributor to these molecular alterations is presented.

https://pubmed.ncbi.nlm.nih.gov/36507225/

The Disease-Modifying Role of Taurine and Its Therapeutic Potential in Coronavirus Disease 2019 (COVID-19)...Taurine is an amino sulfonic acid that is implicated in numerous physiological functions, including the regulation of oxidative stress, which plays an important role in coronavirus disease 2019 (COVID-19), caused by severe acute respiratory syndrome coronavirus 2 (SARS-CoV-2), together with other pathophysiological processes. The recent finding of decreased serum taurine levels in SARS-CoV-2-infected patients, in tandem with its potential modulatory role in COVID-19 due to its antiviral, antioxidant, anti-inflammatory, and vascular-related effects, provides a rationale for considering taurine as a beneficial supplement in patients suffering from COVID-19. Here, we reviewed the potential disease-modifying effects of taurine and combined these with the current knowledge on COVID-19 to clarify the potential role of taurine in this respiratory disease.

https://pubmed.ncbi.nlm.nih.gov/35882777/

Clinical trials on the pharmacological treatment of long COVID: A systematic review...Other supplements such as soy and taurine could be tapped for their roles in regulating TGF-β action directly and indirectly. Lowering TGF-β activity could slow down fibrosis in the lungs or myocardium. l-arginine, the precursor of nitric oxide, could be administered as a supplement with antioxidant effects and vasodilatory properties and potentially improves endothelial function.

https://www.ncbi.nlm.nih.gov/pmc/articles/PMC9878018/

Therapeutic potential of ginger against COVID-19: Is there enough evidence?...In addition to the respiratory system, severe acute respiratory syndrome coronavirus 2 (SARS-CoV-2) strikes other systems, including the digestive, circulatory, urogenital, and even the central nervous system, as its receptor angiotensin-converting enzyme 2 (ACE2) is expressed in various organs, such as lungs, intestine, heart, esophagus, kidneys, bladder, testis, liver, and brain. Different mechanisms, in particular, massive virus replication, extensive apoptosis and necrosis of the lung-related epithelial and endothelial cells, vascular leakage, hyper-inflammatory responses, overproduction of pro-inflammatory mediators, cytokine storm, oxidative stress, downregulation of ACE2, and impairment of the renin-angiotensin system contribute to the COVID-19 pathogenesis. Currently, COVID-19 is a global pandemic with no specific anti-viral treatment. The favorable capabilities of the ginger were indicated in patients suffering from osteoarthritis, neurodegenerative disorders, rheumatoid arthritis, type 2 diabetes, respiratory distress, liver diseases and primary dysmenorrheal. Ginger or its compounds exhibited strong anti-inflammatory and anti-oxidative influences in numerous animal models. This review provides evidence regarding the potential effects of ginger against SARS-CoV-2 infection and highlights its antiviral, anti-inflammatory, antioxidative, and immunomodulatory impacts in an attempt to consider this plant as an alternative therapeutic agent for COVID-19 treatment.

https://www.ncbi.nlm.nih.gov/pmc/articles/PMC8492833/

Role of inositol to improve surfactant functions and reduce IL-6 levels: A potential adjuvant strategy for SARS-CoV-2 pneumonia?...Although the infection can be asymptomatic, several cases develop severe pneumonia and acute respiratory distress syndrome (ARDS) characterized by high levels of pro-inflammatory cytokines, primarily interleukin (IL)-6. Based on available data, the severity of ARDS and serum levels of IL-6 are key determinants for the prognosis. In this scenario, available in vitro and in vivo data suggested that myo-inositol is able to increase the synthesis and function of the surfactant phosphatidylinositol, acting on the phosphoinositide 3-kinase (PI3K)-regulated signaling, with amelioration of both immune system and oxygenation at the bronchoalveolar level. In addition, myo-inositol has been found able to decrease the levels of IL-6 in several experimental settings, due to an effect on the inositol-requiring enzyme 1 (IRE1)-X-box-binding protein 1 (XBP1) and on the signal transducer and activator of transcription 3 (STAT3) pathways. In this scenario, treatment with myo-inositol may be able to reduce IL-6 dependent inflammatory response and improve oxygenation in patients with severe ARDS by SARS-CoV-2. In addition, the action of myo-inositol on IRE1 endonuclease activity may also inhibit the replication of SARS-CoV-2, as was reported for the respiratory syncytial virus. Since the available data are extremely limited, if this potential therapeutic approach will be considered valid in the clinical practice, the necessary future investigations should aim to identify the best dose, administration route (oral, intravenous and/or aerosol nebulization), and cluster(s) of patients which may get beneficial effects from this treatment.

https://www.ncbi.nlm.nih.gov/pmc/articles/PMC7480225/

Medicinal Herbs in the Relief of Neurological, Cardiovascular, and Respiratory Symptoms after COVID-19 Infection A Literature Review...COVID-19 infection causes complications, even in people who have had a mild course of the disease. The most dangerous seem to be neurological ailments: anxiety, depression, mixed anxiety–depressive (MAD) syndromes, and irreversible dementia. These conditions can negatively affect the respiratory system, circulatory system, and heart functioning. We believe that phytotherapy can be helpful in all of these conditions. Clinical trials confirm this possibility. The work presents plant materials (Valeriana officinalis, Melissa officinalis, Passiflora incarnata, Piper methysticum, Humulus lupulus, Ballota nigra, Hypericum perforatum, Rhodiola rosea, Lavandula officinalis, Paullinia cupana, Ginkgo biloba, Murraya koenigii,

Crataegus monogyna and oxyacantha, Hedera helix, Polygala senega, Pelargonium sidoides, Lichen islandicus, Plantago lanceolata) and their dominant compounds (valeranon, valtrate, apigenin, citronellal, isovitexin, isoorientin, methysticin, humulone, farnesene, acteoside, hypericin, hyperforin, biapigenin, rosavidin, salidroside, linalool acetate, linalool, caffeine, ginkgolide, bilobalide, mihanimbine, epicatechin, hederacoside C,α-hederine, presegenin, umckalin, 6,7,8-trixydroxybenzopyranone disulfate, fumaroprotocetric acid, protolichesteric acid, aucubin, acteoside) responsible for their activity. It also shows the possibility of reducing post-COVID-19 neurological, respiratory, and cardiovascular complications, which can affect the functioning of the nervous system.

https://www.ncbi.nlm.nih.gov/pmc/articles/PMC9220793/

Amazonian fruits with potential effects on COVID-19 by inflammaging modulation: A narrative review...The COVID-19 pandemic had a great impact on the mortality of older adults and, chronic non- transmissible diseases (CNTDs) patients, likely previous inflammaging condition that is common in these subjects. It is possible that functional foods could attenuate viral infection conditions such as SARS-CoV-2 (severe acute respiratory syndrome coronavirus 2), the causal agent of COVID-19 pandemic. Previous evidence suggested that some fruits consumed by Amazonian Diet from Pre-Colombian times could present relevant proprieties to decrease of COVID-19 complications such as oxidative-cytokine storm. In this narrative review we identified five potential Amazonian fruits: açai berry (Euterpe oleracea), camu-camu (Myrciaria dubia), cocoa (Theobroma cacao), Brazil nuts (Bertholletia excelsa), and guaraná (Paullinia cupana). Data showed that these Amazonian fruits present antioxidant, anti-inflammatory and other immunomodulatory activities that could attenuate the impact of inflammaging states that potentially decrease the evolution of COVID-19 complications. The evidence compiled here supports the complementary experimental and clinical studies exploring these fruits as nutritional supplement during COVID-19 infection. PRACTICAL APPLICATIONS:

These fruits, in their natural form, are often limited to their region, or exported to other places in the form of frozen pulp or powder. But there are already some companies producing food supplements in the form of capsules, in the form of oils and even functional foods enriched with these fruits. This practice is common in Brazil and tends to expand to the international market.

https://pubmed.ncbi.nlm.nih.gov/36240164/

"Energy drinks may be beneficial for Long COVID patients."

Steven Magee

Coffee

A Google search of 'pubmed 2023 long covid coffee' produced no relevant findings. It appears there is little research being done in this area.

"Coffee is part of my Long COVID supplementing protocol."

Steven Magee

Tea

The medicinal value of tea drinking in the management of COVID-19...Corona Virus Disease 2019 (COVID-19) is presently the largest international public health event, individuals infected by the virus not only have symptoms such as fever, dry cough, and lung infection at the time of onset, but also possibly have sequelae in the cardiovascular system, respiratory system, nervous system, mental health and other aspects. However, numerous studies have depicted that the active ingredients in tea show good antiviral effects and can treat various diseases by regulating multiple pathways, and the therapeutic effects are associated with the categories of chemical components in tea. In this review, the differences in the content of key active ingredients in different types of tea are summarized. In addition, we also highlighted their effects on COVID-19 and connected sequelae, further demonstrating the possibility of developing a formulation for the prevention and treatment of COVID-19 and its sequelae through tea extracts. We have a tendency to suggest forestalling and treating COVID-19 and its sequelae through scientific tea drinking.

https://pubmed.ncbi.nlm.nih.gov/36647394/

Green Tea Consumption and the COVID-19 Omicron Pandemic Era: Pharmacology and Epidemiology...In spite of the development of numerous vaccines for the prevention of COVID-19 and the approval of several drugs for its treatment, there is still a great need for effective and inexpensive therapies against this disease. Previously, we showed that green tea and tea catechins interfere with coronavirus replication as well as coronavirus 3CL protease activity, and also showed lower COVID-19 morbidity and mortality in countries with higher green tea consumption. However, it is not clear whether green tea is still effective against the newer SARS-CoV-2 variants including omicron. It is also not known whether higher green tea consumption continues to contribute to lower COVID-19 morbidity and mortality now that vaccination rates in many countries are high. Here, we attempted to update the information regarding green tea in relation to COVID-19. Using pharmacological and ecological approaches, we found that EGCG as well as green tea inhibit the activity of the omicron variant 3CL protease efficiently, and there continues to be pronounced differences in COVID-19 morbidity and mortality between groups of countries with high and low green tea consumption as of December 6, 2022. These results collectively suggest that green tea continues to be effective against COVID-19 despite the new omicron variants and increased vaccination.

https://pubmed.ncbi.nlm.nih.gov/36984007/

Potential of green tea EGCG in neutralizing SARS-CoV-2 Omicron variant with greater tropism toward the upper respiratory tract...Background: COVID-19 due to SARS-CoV-2 infection has had an enormous adverse impact on global public health. As the COVID-19 pandemic evolves, the WHO declared several variants of concern (VOCs), including Alpha, Beta, Gamma, Delta, and Omicron. Compared with earlier variants, Omicron, now a dominant lineage, exhibits characteristics of enhanced transmissibility, tropism shift toward the upper respiratory tract, and attenuated disease severity. The robust transmission of Omicron despite attenuated disease severity still poses a great challenge for pandemic control. Under this circumstance, its tropism shift may be utilized for discovering effective preventive approaches. Scope and approach: This review aims to estimate the potential of green tea epigallocatechin gallate (EGCG), the most potent antiviral catechin, in neutralizing SARS-CoV-2 Omicron variant, based on current knowledge concerning EGCG distribution in tissues and Omicron tropism. Key findings and conclusions: EGCG has a low bioavailability. Plasma EGCG levels are in the range of submicromolar concentrations following green tea drinking, or reach at most low μM concentrations after pharmacological intervention. Nonetheless, its levels in the upper respiratory tract could reach concentrations as high as tens or even hundreds of μM following green tea consumption or pharmacological intervention. An approach for delivering sufficiently high concentrations of EGCG in the pharynx has been developed. Convincing data have demonstrated that EGCG at tens to hundreds of μM can dramatically neutralize SARS-CoV-2 and effectively eliminate SARS-CoV-2-induced cytopathic effects and plaque formation. Thus, EGCG, which exhibits hyperaccumulation in the upper respiratory tract, deserves closer investigation as an antiviral in the current global battle against COVID-19, given Omicron's greater tropism toward the upper respiratory tract.

https://pubmed.ncbi.nlm.nih.gov/36594074/

Recuperative herbal formula Jing Si maintains vasculature permeability balance, regulates inflammation and assuages concomitants of "Long-Covid"...Coronavirus disease 2019 (COVID-19) is a worldwide health threat that has long-term effects on the patients and there is currently no efficient cure prescribed for the treatment and the prolonging effects. Traditional Chinese medicines (TCMs) have been reported to exert therapeutic effect against COVID-19. In this study, the therapeutic effects of Jing Si herbal tea (JSHT) against COVID-19 infection and associated long-term effects were evaluated in different in vitro and in vivo models. The anti-inflammatory effects of JSHT were studied in lipopolysaccharide (LPS)-stimulated RAW 264.7 cells and in Omicron pseudotyped virus-induced acute lung injury model. The effect of JSHT on cellular stress was determined in HK-2 proximal tubular cells and H9c2 cardiomyoblasts. The therapeutic benefits of JSHT on anhedonia and depression symptoms associated with long COVID were evaluated in mice models for unpredictable chronic mild stress (UCMS). JSHT inhibited the NF-ƙB activities, and significantly reduced LPS-induced expression of TNFα, COX-2, NLRP3 inflammasome, and HMGB1. JSHT was also found to significantly suppress the production of NO by reducing iNOS expression in LPS-stimulated RAW 264.7 cells. Further, the protective effects of JSHT on lung tissue were confirmed based on mitigation of lung injury, repression in TMRRSS2 and HMGB-1 expression and reduction of cytokine storm in the Omicron pseudotyped virus-induced acute lung injury model. JSHT treatment in UCMS models also relieved chronic stress and combated depression symptoms. The results therefore show that JSHT attenuates the cytokine storm by repressing NF-κB cascades and provides the protective functions against symptoms associated with long COVID-19 infection.

https://pubmed.ncbi.nlm.nih.gov/37116351/

"Drinking tea has long been known for its medicinal benefits."

Steven Magee

Hydration

Dietary Recommendations for Post-COVID-19 Syndrome...

At the beginning of the coronavirus disease (COVID-19) pandemic, global efforts focused on containing the spread of the virus and avoiding contagion. Currently, it is evident that health professionals should deal with the overall health status of COVID-19 survivors. Indeed, novel findings have identified post-COVID-19 syndrome, which is characterized by malnutrition, loss of fat-free mass, and low-grade inflammation. In addition, the recovery might be complicated by persistent functional impairment (i.e., fatigue and muscle weakness, dysphagia, appetite loss, and taste/smell alterations) as well as psychological distress. Therefore, the appropriate evaluation of nutritional status (assessment of dietary intake, anthropometrics, and body composition) is one of the pillars in the management of these patients. On the other hand, personalized dietary recommendations represent the best strategy to ensure recovery. Therefore, this review aimed to collect available evidence on the role of nutrients and their supplementation in post-COVID-19 syndrome to provide a practical guideline to nutritionists to tailor dietary interventions for patients recovering from COVID-19 infections...adequate hydration (30 mL/kg actual body weight) is important for the complete recovery of patients with post-COVID-19 syndrome. Therefore, these patients should increase their daily fluid intake (2.5–3 L/day) by consuming water, milk, fruit juice, broth, sports drinks, coffee, and tea.

https://www.ncbi.nlm.nih.gov/pmc/articles/PMC8954128/

"Optimal hydration is needed when recovering from Long COVID."

Steven Magee

Altitude Hypersensitivity

Coronavirus damages the lungs and many people have been diagnosed with small airways disease after developing long COVID. Damaged lungs can develop pressure sensitivities. This may bring on altitude and weather sensitivities. A low or high pressure weather system passing through your area may make you sick! Changing altitude by flying, driving, vacationing, hiking or skiing may make you sick. Living at altitude may keep you in a permanent state of sickness from hypoxic altitude sickness health issues. If you are on a CPAP or BiPAP machine, these may may you sickly from the pressurized air they feed to you! If you have had coronavirus, you should be watching for these pressure related health issues!

When I discovered I had altitude hypersensitivity and I was developing altitude sickness at just 1,000 feet, my initial thought was it may be a life long condition. However, experiments with nutritional supplements in combination with regular altitude exposures were revealing the condition was reducing in severity.

I had a lucky break in this research and that came from my ex-girlfriend. During the relationship, she had been complaining of a lack of sex drive and a lack of interest in sex. She believed she was in menopause. As such, I bought her a menopause support supplement called "Amberen" that was supposed to reduce the symptoms of menopause. However, she refused to take it.

Wondering what to do with the Amberen I now owned, I looked up the formulation and found it had no female hormones in it. It was just a nutritional support supplement. I could see no reason why a man could not take it. A daily dose of Amberen contains a 400 mg blend of the following:

- Ammonium Succinate.
- Calcium Disuccinate.
- Monosodium L-Glutamate.

- Glycine.

- Magnesium Disuccinate.

- Zinc Difumarate.

- Tocopheryl Acetate.

The manufacturer states: *"Amberen contains a proprietary blend of bioactive antioxidants, amino acids, minerals and vitamin E."*

So I started to take it in June 2022. A week after taking the Amberen, I did an altitude test. I took my body up from 600 feet above sea level to 4,024 feet and much to my surprise noticed no symptoms that could make a diagnosis of altitude hypersensitivity. A few days later I took my body from 140 feet above sea level to 6,632 feet and again saw no symptoms that could make a diagnosis of altitude hypersensitivity.

This was the first time this had occurred during altitude testing. The Amberen had changed the body chemistry. I had noticed nerve pains in my face accompanied by twitching since I had been taking this supplement, so something was changing in the body regarding the nervous system.

The Amberen had fixed things! Why was this? Because I was age 52, I was in "Manopause". Manopause is the male equivalent of the female menopause. Just like aged females, the hormones also change in men after forty years of age. Hormone decline occurs in both sexes after age forty. But was there any evidence it could be the Amberen?

I took a look at the Amberen website and found this statement: *"Glycine: An amino acid involved in the processes regulating brain-cell activity. In combination with magnesium, it makes brain mitochondria more resistant to low-oxygen conditions (hypoxia), which, in turn, results in the normalization of the psycho-emotional balance in the body."*

https://amberen.com/am-ingredients

So one of the ingredients of Amberen is a known treatment for hypoxia! I was right! Increasing altitude causes hypoxia and glycine treats it. To confirm the information was correct on the Amberen website, I did an internet search on "glycine altitude" and found numerous articles about its beneficial effects at altitude.

After one month of taking Amberen:

- Regular altitude testing from sea level up to 6,632 feet was showing no evidence of altitude hypersensitivity.

- The side effects were:
    - Nerve pains in my face.
    - Facial muscles twitching.
    - Insomnia.
    - Mild headaches.
    - Mild heart pains.
    - All side effects subsided after one month of Amberen administration.

Amberen treats altitude hypersensitivity. Altitude hypersensitivity at 1,000 feet returned during minimum supplement testing and this indicated it was one of the removed supplements that was causing it. Reviewing my notes indicated that it had followed the removal of Acetyl-L-Carnitine HCl. Taking L-Carnitine L-Tartrate at 500mg daily cleared up the altitude hypersensitivity.

Why did I switch from Acetyl-L-Carnitine HCl to L-Carnitine L-Tartrate? I could not purchase Acetyl-L-Carnitine HCl at the time, due to the COVID-19 pandemic shortages. L-Carnitine L-Tartrate was the closest thing to it that was available for purchase.

The question arose of what was the minimum amount of supplements needed to prevent altitude hypersensitivity from occurring? I removed all supplements with the exception of

Amberen and L-Carnitine L-Tartrate and continued to be free of altitude hypersensitivity. I did see some adverse reactions to L-Carnitine L-Tartrate as I raised the dose to 500 mg 4 times daily (total 2,000 mg daily):

- Day 1: No symptoms.

- Day 2: Hungry all day long and overeating.

- Day 3: Fatigued all day long and stayed in bed. Low appetite.

- Day 4: Mating cycle was triggered during morning sleep. Woke up at sunrise. Headache all day long. Stayed in bed most of the day.

- Day 5: Milder headache and lethargic. In bed in the afternoon with headache. The headache seemed to increase as I was taking the four doses of L-Carnitine L-Tartrate during the day. Right earache during the evening that subsided by bedtime.

- Day 6: Mild headache that subsided by lunchtime. Afternoon fatigue. Altitude test to 4,024 feet. No symptoms of altitude hypersensitivity. Sore right knee joint when walking in the evening.

- Day 7: Woke up energized. Fatigue onset as the day progressed that did not respond to caffeine. Hungry in the evening and overeating.

- Day 8: Woke up at sunrise. Fatigued and exhibiting confusion. Altitude test to 6,632 feet. No symptoms of altitude hypersensitivity. Ears popping and skull pains.

- Day 9: Feeling fine.

The dose was raised to what the manufacturer recommended, as I was concerned that I may not be taking enough of it to fully treat the altitude hypersensitivity. Based on the above symptoms, there was a profound response to the increased dosing which I took as an indication that a deficiency was being corrected in the body.

I removed the Amberen to see if the L-Carnitine L-Tartrate could treat altitude hypersensitivity on its own.

Research into L-Carnitine L-Tartrate indicated that 3,000 mg is considered the safe level of maximum dosing in adults. Given the profound reactions I was having to it, I decided to do a couple of weeks at 3 doses daily of 1,000 mg. The following reactions were seen at the maximum dosing level:

- Day 1: Insomnia until 1 am.

- Day 2: Woke up fatigued. Coffee cleared it. Had good energy levels and concentration.

- Day 3: Had good energy levels and concentration.

- Day 4: Fatigued PM.

- Day 5: Feeling fine. Altitude test to 2,000 feet. No symptoms of altitude hypersensitivity.

- Day 6: Feeling fine.

- Day 7 to 10: Started to develop mild headaches.

- Day 11: Altitude test to 4,024 feet. Mild headache that progressed into severe headache at altitude. Showing increasing confusion during the drive. Started Amberen to treat the headache and confusion. Both subsided during sleep.

- Day 12: At 140 feet above sea level. Fatigued in the morning that responded to caffeine.

- Day 13: Altitude test to 6,632 feet. Feeling normal. Mild headache during altitude exposure. Cleared up at sea level in Kona. No further issues on the drive home at 1,000 to 2,000 feet. Slept at 600 feet.

- Day 14: Mild skull pains.

- Day 15: Back to normal.

Removing Amberen did cause altitude hypersensitivity to return. It was also accompanied by headaches. Taking the Amberen cleared up both conditions. It appears the altitude exposure is needed for nutritional absorption throughout the body, including the brain.

There appears to be two supplements needed to keep altitude hypersensitivity treated once it has been cleared and that is:

- L-Carnitine L-Tartrate at 500 mg to 3,000 mg daily.
  - Bulk Supplements.
- Amberen.
  - Biogix, Inc.

L-Carnitine and Amberen were working together to clear up the altitude hypersensitivity. There is an interaction taking place between them and one does not work without the other.

I have remained free of most food intolerance using only L-Carnitine L-Tartrate. Mental and physical health were good. Energy levels were good.

Regarding the rest of the supplements, it seems they reduce the altitude hypersensitivity, but they do not fully clear it up like the L-Carnitine and Amberen do. Given the rest of the supplements improve sex, it appears they are treating deficiencies within the body.

The key suspected ingredients that treat altitude hypersensitivity were L-Carnitine and glycine. Research revealed a supplement that had both of these in it called "Glycine Propionyl-L-Carnitine (GPLC)". I purchased the following GPLC products:

- Carlyle GPLC Supplement 1250mg.
  - Propionyl-L-Carnitine 824 mg.
  - Glycine 282 mg.
  - CoQ10 60 mg.

- VitaMonk GlycoTrax.
  - ○ Glycine Propionyl-L-Carnitine 1,000 mg.

L-Carnitine and Amberen were removed and were replaced by GPLC. My body remained free of altitude hypersensitivity during altitude tests. I took GPLC for three months and did not see altitude hypersensitivity return during that time.

There was a notable difference in the GPLC supplements. Carlyle GPLC was unstable and would degrade after opening the supplement container. When I would put it in my pill box, by the end of a week the Carlyle GPLC capsules would be degrading. After a couple of months in the pill bottle, they were unusable. I threw the last few capsules I had away. No such issues were observed with VitaMonk GlycoTrax. The Carlyle GPLC appeared to be the better GPLC supplement for treating altitude hypersensitivity and this reflected its higher level of GPLC.

These are my conclusions about treating my altitude hypersensitivity:

- Low protein organic diet.

- Base nutritional supplements are L-Carnitine and glycine.

- Optimized nutrition through appropriate supplementation and diet.

There is currently no known cure for altitude hypersensitivity, it appears to be a lifelong treatment. It may be arising in the general population from flying, mountain activities, living at altitude, lung damage, man-made environmental changes, climate change and new bacteria and viruses.

"I was surprised at how simple the treatment for Altitude Hypersensitivity was."

Steven Magee

Altitude Sickness

There are five different ranges of altitudes that altitude sickness falls into:

1. Sea Level:
   ○ A damaged body in a state of altitude sickness at sea level.
   ○ Acclimatization never occurs.

2. Altitude Hypersensitivity:
   ○ Above sea level to 4,900 feet.
   ○ Acclimatization only occurs below the "Altitude Hypersensitivity Threshold" where symptoms are not observed.

3. High Altitude:
   ○ 4,900 to 11,500 feet.

4. Very High Altitude:
   ○ 11,500 to 18,000 ft.

5. Extreme Altitude:
   ○ Above 18,000 ft.

Hypoxia ties altitude sickness, COVID-19 and long COVID together. The symptoms to look out for are:

- Headache.
- Confusion.
- Fatigue.
- Stomach illness.
- Dizziness.

- Sleep disturbance.

- Central sleep apnea.

- Exertion may aggravate the symptoms.

If you are experiencing any of the above symptoms, you may need to move to a rural sea level area to recover. If you are unable to move, then altitude sickness supplements and/or treatments may be able to improve your health. More information can be found in the book "Toxic Altitude" by Steven Magee.

"After my flu-like illness, I was telling the doctors my progressing sickness felt like Altitude Sickness!"

Steven Magee

Pandemic Supplements 1

This was the first supplementation system I developed for treating my long COVID symptoms:

Steven Magee takes daily:

- Daily multivitamin.
  - Kirkland Signature.
- Calcium citrate, magnesium and zinc.
  - Kirkland Signature.
- Wild alaskan salmon oil 1,000 mg.
  - Pure Alaska Omega.
- Betaine HCI, pepsin and genetian bitters.
  - Doctor's best.
- Vitamin B12 5,000 mcg.
  - Kirkland Signature.
- Vitamin C 1,000 mg.
  - Kirkland Signature.
- Vitamin D 10,000 IU.
  - Carlyle.
- Alpha Lipoic Acid 300 mg.
  - Puritan's Pride.
- Folic acid 400 mcg.
  - Sundown.
- Iron 65 mg.
  - Nature Made.

- Creatine Monohydrate 3 g.
  - Now Sports.
- Amino acid drink 10 g.
  - Essential amino energy by Optimum Nutrition.
- L-Citrulline 6 g.
  - Bulk Supplements.
- L-Lysine-HCL 1.5 g.
  - Bulk Supplements.
- Acetyl-L-Carnitine HCI 750 mg.
  - Jacked Factory.
- L-Arginine 500 mg.
  - Jacked Factory.
- Amberen.
  - Biogix, Inc.
- Testosterone Support one capsule.
  - Weider Prime.
- Extreme Test one capsule.
  - Influx Inspire.
- Breakfast is a pot of coffee (12 cups - 60 ounces) slowly consumed between sunrise and noon.
  - Kirkland Signature whole bean french roast coffee.
  - Kirkland Signature organic coffee creamer french vanilla flavored.

The iron tablet can be replaced with an iron fish, which may be more effective in the long term. "Kirkland" branded products are obtained at Costco.

The supplements are taken at breakfast, around 7 am. Missing a dose of the supplements generally causes sleepiness and fatigue to occur by 3 pm onward. This can be offset by taking the missed supplements. If the missed supplements are not taken until the next morning, then a progressive feeling of sickness will occur during the night. Taking the supplements the next morning clears the sickness.

Regarding food intake, I only drink liquids in the morning until noon. Breakfast is coffee and creamer. Lunch and dinner are solids and they are eaten between noon and 6pm. Food and drink intake is as follows:

- Sunrise: Wake up and spend 30 minutes outdoors.

- Morning: Take supplements with coffee and creamer.

- Noon: Start eating solids for lunch.

- 5pm: Solids dinner.

- 6pm: Start fasting, drink water only if needed.

- Sunset: Watch sunset for light absorption into the body to prepare it for sleep.

- Once the onset of tiredness takes place, go to bed with the curtains open for starlight, planet and moonlight exposures during sleep. The head of the bed needs to be under the window so that nighttime light can shine onto the face.

- Food fasting starts at 6pm and goes through to sunrise the next day.

- Liquids fast is typically 12 hours long.

- Liquids are only consumed for approximately 12 hours per day.

- Solids fast is typically 18 hours long.

- Solids are only eaten for 6 hours per day.

The supplements need to be taken in conjunction with daily outdoor exercise. That exercise should be a mix of cardio and muscle building exercise that is done for at least an hour. Vigorous swimming, lifting weights and/or cycling hills are effective. Regular sex is an excellent cardio exercise.

Long term testing over several months revealed the side effects of this supplement plan:

- Nerve damage at 9,200 feet occurred after an altitude test. (May not be related to the supplements.)
- Sore knees.
- Cramping in the right foot and right hand.

"Nutritional supplements had far more beneficial effects than any of the prescription drugs."

Steven Magee

Minimum Supplements

One of the things I like to do is find out what are the minimum amount of supplements I need to take to maintain improved health. As such, I removed some of supplements I thought were non-essential at the time to see if I would continue in good health. The following were removed in August 2022:

- Daily multivitamin.
  - Kirkland Signature.
- Wild alaskan salmon oil 1,000 mg.
  - Pure Alaska Omega.
- Betaine HCI, pepsin and genetian bitters.
  - Doctor's best.
- Creatine Monohydrate 3 g.
  - Now Sports.
- Acetyl-L-Carnitine HCI 750 mg.
  - Jacked Factory.
- L-Arginine 500 mg.
  - Jacked Factory.

I did see an adverse reaction to removing Creatine Monohydrate. It caused severe sensitivity in my teeth, it was so severe that I could only eat liquid foods after five days of not taking it. The sensitive teeth subsided after two weeks. Stopping Acetyl-L-Carnitine HCI did bring on sensitive teeth for a couple of days.

The reduced supplements did have a negative effect on sexual functioning and reintroducing the full range of supplements fixed it. I had better sex and sexual stamina on the full range of supplements.

"It is important to experiment with supplements to verify you actually need to take them. Taking a non-essential supplement is just wasting your money."

Steven Magee

Pandemic Supplements 2

This supplement plan was developed to eliminate the knee pains that the first one was causing. It was suspected the knee pains were coming from supplement toxicity, so known toxic supplements were removed. Some supplements that were thought not to be needed anymore were also removed. The removed supplements did clear up the knee pains.

Steven Magee takes daily:

- Daily multivitamin.
  - Kirkland Signature.
- Calcium citrate, magnesium and zinc.
  - Kirkland Signature.
- Wild alaskan salmon oil 1,000 mg.
  - Pure Alaska Omega.
- Vitamin C 1,000 mg.
  - Kirkland Signature.
- Amino acid drink 10 g.
  - Essential amino energy by Optimum Nutrition.
- L-Citrulline 6 g.
  - Bulk Supplements.
- L-Lysine-HCL 1.5 g.
  - Bulk Supplements.
- Acetyl-L-Carnitine HCI 750 mg.
  - Jacked Factory.
- L-Arginine 500 mg.

- ○ Jacked Factory.
- Amberen.
  - ○ Biogix, Inc.
- Testosterone Support one capsule.
  - ○ Weider Prime.
- Extreme Test one capsule.
  - ○ Influx Inspire.
- Breakfast is a pot of coffee (12 cups - 60 ounces) slowly consumed between sunrise and noon.
  - ○ Kirkland Signature whole bean french roast coffee.
  - ○ Kirkland Signature organic coffee creamer french vanilla flavored.
- Kidney Cleanse as needed.
  - ○ Dr. Bo.

Sexual performance was excellent with long lasting sex sessions. It was further improved by doubling the dose of the testosterone boosting supplements.

A kidney cleanse was performed during this supplement protocol due to recognizing that the kidneys were involved in the amino acid deficiencies I have.

"It is important to know which supplements you are taking are associated with toxicity to the human."

Steven Magee

Pandemic Supplements 3

This set of supplements was for improved nail and skin growth. I was still having fungal toenail growth and I was suspicious the fungal infection was systemic. I had a history of skin tags on my body after my flu-like illness that brought on long COVID symptoms. Research indicated the most effective treatment for fungal nails was an oral anti-fungal medication. This set of supplements was developed to attempt to counteract a systemic fungal infection.

The Amberen and L-Carnitine were removed, as I wanted to see if they could be replaced by GPLC to treat altitude hypersensitivity. Testing went well with GPLC and it does effectively treat altitude hypersensitivity.

The amino acid powders were removed to make it easier to travel. Traveling through airports with white powdered amino acids may flag you up to TSA as a suspected drugs dealer. I have had this experience in Kona airport in Hawaii and it is unpleasant! They tested all of the powders for drugs and it delayed me going through TSA! It was all done in front of the passengers going through the TSA area, so the passengers know what is going on. I got some strange looks from passengers once I was inside the airport gate area!

Two weeks after the amino acid powders were removed, the food sensitivities came back. I was getting very sleepy after some large evening meals. I introduced a 1,000 mg tablet of L-Arginine daily and within a few days, the food sensitivities were reduced but not completely gone. Adding Citrulline to it brought on headaches but did not clear up the food sensitivities. I happened to drink a can of "Monster Energy" with my morning supplements that I had got free with a purchase at a store. This completely cleared the headaches up!

Why would "Monster Energy" clear up the headaches? It has some extra supplements in it that were not in my regular daily supplements:

- Taurine.

- Panax Ginseng.

- L-Carnitine L-Tartrate.

- Guarana.

- Other ingredients.

There is something in this drink that interacted with my supplements to clear up the headaches. It required just one 16 fluid ounces can to be taken with the morning supplements. I suspect the "Monster Energy" was acting as a catalyst that increased or altered the pre-existing chemistry of my supplements. It triggered a beneficial reaction that only required one dose. Once the reaction had occurred, my existing supplements were sufficient at preventing headaches and they did not return. The ingredients in "Monster Energy" has commonality with some of the supplements that were used in the pandemic supplement protocols described in this book.

Food intolerance was still present in the evening after eating a large evening meal, bringing on tiredness and sleepiness. Mental functioning was beginning to decline and I was starting to feel weird brain functioning. It seemed the travel supplements were not fully treating the nutritional deficiencies I had.

The home where I was staying had a canister of "Amino Energy" and decided to start taking the full recommended dose of six scoops daily. I would take two scoops as soon as I woke up, another two scoops mid-morning and the final two scoops at lunchtime. This cleared up the food intolerance and brain functioning issues after one week.

Adjusting to six scoops daily of "Amino Energy" did bring on the following conditions in the first week:

- Nerve pains.

- Dreams.

Once the adjustment took place, the symptoms subsided and I was feeling good again! Lots of energy daily, no fatigue and good mental functioning.

The "Amino Energy" powder was replaced with amino acid tablets called "Amino Acid Complex 3000mg" by Horbaach. There was a mild headache reaction after several days that lasted for a day and cleared with sleep. I did get a brief period where I could remember dreaming for a few days. I remained free of symptoms and had developed a tablet based amino acid supplementation protocol that worked for me.

I stopped taking the multivitamin and replaced it with B-complex. This was due to being on the multivitamin for almost a year and I wanted to take a break from it.

I decided to replace the calcium citrate, magnesium and zinc with just magnesium and to increase the dose. This was due to seeing an increase in sleeping oxygen events. I took the magnesium up to 250 mg from 80 mg daily.

The supplement system did not feel quite right, so a little research on it revealed it was very similar to what is being used to treat autistic children. Zinc is a big feature of that treatment. As such, I raised the zinc levels by adding a 50 mg zinc tablet daily. The reviews of the zinc supplement were showing 50 mg daily was well tolerated by most people.

Memory and confusion had slowly increased during developing this supplement protocol and had subsided once it had been fully developed.

The increased levels of the amino acids in the prior supplement protocols appear to improve sexual functioning. Adding in the zinc brought on morning erections and improved things. Sexual functioning waned during development of this supplement protocol before normalizing once completed.

Steven Magee takes daily:

- Magnesium Citrate 250 mg.
  - Nature Made.
- Zinc 50 mg.
  - Nature's Bounty.
- Wild alaskan salmon oil 1,000 mg.
  - Pure Alaska Omega.
- Super B complex with vitamin C one tablet.
  - CVS Health.
- Vitamin C 2,000 mg.
  - Kirkland Signature.
- Vitamin E 180 mg.
  - Kirkland Signature.
  - For external use. Paint one capsule onto affected fungal nails and skin daily after showering.
- Vitamin E 1,440 mg.
  - Kirkland Signature.
- Biotin 10,000 mcg.
  - Bronson.
- GPLC two capsules.
  - Carlyle.
- L-Arginine & L-Citrulline one tablet.
  - Amazing Nutrition.
- Amino Acid Complex three tablets.
  - Horbaach.
- Testosterone Support one capsule.

- ○ Weider Prime.
- Extreme Test one capsule.
  - ○ Influx Inspire.
- Organic greek yogurt plain one tablespoon with each meal.
  - ○ Kirkland.
- Breakfast is a pot of coffee (12 cups - 60 ounces) slowly consumed between sunrise and noon.
  - ○ Kirkland Signature whole bean french roast coffee.
  - ○ Full cream milk.
- "Monster Energy" 16 fluid ounces if needed.
  - ○ Monster Energy Company.

Sore shoulders and neck were observed in the first few weeks of taking this supplement combination and it slowly subsided. It was suspected to be the adjustment to the high dose of vitamin E. The area of my upper back and neck soreness were consistent with the area associated with Kyphosis. Kyphosis is an abnormally excessive convex curvature of the spine as it occurs in the thoracic and sacral regions.

Stools were looser on this supplement protocol and it was thought to be the anti-fungal properties of vitamin E that were affecting the contents of the digestive tract. Daily morning defecations were easy and pleasant.

Improved nail and hair growth was observed during the time I have been taking this supplement protocol. At three months into high dosing of vitamin E I was not noticing any side effects or toxicity associated with it. Vitamin E toxicity showed up in me during the fourth month of high daily dosing. It was a sensation of not feeling well with brain fog and I was making driving mistakes. Pulse oximeter testing showed that my heart rate was elevated by about 30 beats per minute (BPM) more than normal at 95 BPM while sitting. Stopping the vitamin E cleared the toxicity and restored the natural heart rate. Withdrawal symptoms were mild and included some insomnia, dizziness and aches and pains in the following weeks.

Zinc toxicity showed up in me during the fifth month of high daily dosing. It was disturbed sleep patterns, insomnia, mild headaches, sensitive teeth, lower back pains and short term memory issues. Stopping the zinc supplement fixed things in a few days after some fatigue and tiredness from withdrawing the zinc supplement.

I was free of food intolerance symptoms and could eat a normal diet. I was not avoiding any food types. I could eat a huge pepperoni pizza from Costco without any issues.

This supplement system produced the highest energy levels. I was very alert and capable on it. A lot of jobs were getting done on my home!

After I wrapped up research on pandemic supplements 3, my supply of GPLC ran out. I noticed glycine was contained within the amino acid complex tablets and all I had to do was add in the L-Carnitine to replace the GPLC. I had L-Carnitine L-Tartrate from previous testing and I replaced the GPLC with it at a single 2 g daily dose. My body remained free of Altitude Hypersensitivity.

Coffee was replaced with tea, as I had been drinking coffee for over a year and wanted to take a break from it. My body remained in comparable condition on the tea.

"Traveling through airports with white powders may get you flagged by TSA as a potential drugs dealer!"

Steven Magee

Supplement Overdose Symptoms

During developing pandemic supplements I did experience symptoms of supplement overdosing:

- Changed taste – coffee did not taste right, regardless of brand.

- Aching joints.

- Not feeling well.

- Brain fog.

- Driving mistakes.

- Elevated heart rate.

- Disturbed sleep patterns.

- Insomnia.

- Mild headaches.

- Sensitive teeth.

- Lower back pains.

- Short term memory issues.

It is important when taking supplements to research the side effects of them to know when you may be displaying them. Changing my pandemic supplement protocol from 1 to 2 did eliminate the sore joints. My taste remained changed and I expect that will not rectify itself until I reduce my supplements to a maintenance dose of just what is essential for me.

The changed taste had coincided with a virus that I had while traveling around the USA in October and November 2022. The virus did not test positive for COVID-19, although the symptoms were similar. I had a couple of days of mild flu-like symptoms with lung pains during sleeping. It cleared up and the only symptom I was left with was all types of coffee tasting bland. It all tasted the same to me regardless of brand or roast.

Supplement symptoms typically subside in the weeks after removing the supplement that caused them. It is common to see withdrawal symptoms during that time.

"When taking nutritional supplements, it is important to know which ones have toxicity associated with them."

Steven Magee

Medical Tests

You should be aware that nutritional supplementing can affect the results of numerous medical tests. It can hide medical conditions from detection. Some of the test results known to be affected by nutritional supplements are:

- Thyroid hormone.

- Vitamin D.

- Calcium.

- Prostate specific-antigen (PSA).

- Hepatitis B.

- Hepatitis C.

- COVID-19.

- Heart attack.

- Bone density scans.

- Stool.

- Cardiac diseases.

- Endocrine disorders.

- Cancers.

- Anemias.

- Kidney disease.

- Infectious diseases.

The higher the doses of nutritional supplements are, the more likely they are to interfere with medical tests. Known supplements that cause medical test problems are:

- Riboflavin (B2).
- Biotin (B7).
- Niacin.
- Vitamin B12.
- Vitamin C.
- Vitamin E.
- Calcium.
- Iron.
- L-tryptophan.
- St. John's wort.
- 5-HTP.

Other things that are known to affect medical test results are:

- Some foods.
- Some drinks.
- Intense physical activity.
- Sunburn.
- Colds
- Infections.
- Having sex.
- Some medications or drugs.
- Lack of sleep.
- Dehydration.

You should discuss your nutritional supplement intake with your doctor prior to ordering medical tests. You should query abnormal test results that may have been adversely affected by nutritional supplements. Both "false-positive" and "false-negative" test results are known to occur.

"Nutritional supplements may give you false or inaccurate results on medical laboratory tests."

Steven Magee

Supplement Toxicity

The following supplements are well known to have the ability to cause toxicity in the human:

- An excess of vitamin B6.
- Fat soluble vitamins A, D, E, and K.
- Iron tablets.

When taking supplements and noticing the onset of unusual health issues, it is wise to review the toxicity of the supplements you are taking.

"Supplement toxicity in me was causing sore knees. I removed the suspected supplements and the sore knees disappeared!"

Steven Magee

Long COVID Case Studies

Corona With Lyme: A Long COVID Case Study...The case presented describes the three-year arc of a previously healthy 26-year-old female medical student from initial infection and induction of long COVID symptomology to near-total remission of the disease. In doing so, the course of this unique post-viral illness and the trials and errors of myriad treatment options will be chronologized, thereby contributing to the continued demand for understanding this mystifying disease...A previously healthy 26-year-old female medical student living in New York, NY, was one of the first of her colleagues to be symptomatically infected with the then-novel coronavirus, SARS-CoV-2, in March 2020...The patient remained asymptomatic until mid-July 2020 when she abruptly began experiencing the symptoms, which eventually contributed to her long COVID diagnosis. At this initiation, the patient described a sudden and unprovoked burning sensation starting from her forehead and radiating through her entire scalp and down her neck. The sensation persisted for several hours before eventually dissipating and being followed by intense frontotemporal headaches, chest tightness with some dyspnea, palpitations and tachycardia with anxiety, dizziness with episodes of near-syncope on sitting or standing, and blurred vision. In the days following, the aforementioned symptoms would resume upon waking each morning and persist throughout the day. They were eventually coupled with significant fatigue, mild cognitive impairment or "brain fog" with impaired focus and memory recall, loss of appetite, diarrhea, uncharacteristic heat intolerance, and diffuse myalgias. The final symptom to appear during this cascade was severe, right-sided shoulder joint and/or muscle pain with radiations to the neck and right upper extremity, which led the patient to seek treatment...In January 2021, the patient completed the two-dose Moderna mRNA COVID-19 vaccination course and noted moderate improvements in her fatigue and brain fog in the first 24 hours following her first dose. Her headaches and scalp allodynia eventually receded as well nearly six months later in

August 2021. To date, the patient identifies as having made a full recovery from long COVID and only endorses residual blurred vision managed with a stronger vision prescription and reduced but continued oligomenorrhea and hypoglycemic sensitivity managed with diet, exercise, and metformin treatment. She has since been reinfected twice with SARS-CoV-2 in July 2022 and January 2023 and received molnupiravir for the first of these two reinfections but spontaneously recovered both times without relapse of any of her long COVID symptoms.

https://www.ncbi.nlm.nih.gov/pmc/articles/PMC10122830/

"Smart people learn from the experiences of others."

Steven Magee

Long COVID Treatments

Depression and brain fog as long-COVID mental health consequences: Difficult, complex and partially successful treatment of a 72-year-old patient-A case report...SARS-CoV-2 (COVID-19) infection can result in long-term health consequences i.e., long COVID. The clinical manifestations of long COVID include depression, anxiety, brain fog with cognitive dysfunction, memory issues, and fatigue. These delayed effects of COVID-19 occur in up to 30% of people who have had an acute case of COVID-19. In this case report, a 72-year-old, fully vaccinated patient without pre-existing somatic or mental illnesses, or other relevant risk factors was diagnosed with long COVID. Nine months following an acute COVID-19 infection, the patient's depressive symptoms improved, but memory and concentration difficulties persisted, and the patient remains unable to resume work. These long-term symptoms are possibly linked to micro-hemorrhages detected during examinations of the patient's brain following COVID-19 infection. Patient treatment was complex, and positive results were attained via antidepressants and non-drug therapies e.g., art, music, drama, dance and movement therapy, physiotherapy, occupational therapy, and psychotherapy.

https://pubmed.ncbi.nlm.nih.gov/37032935/

"There is little information on how to treat Long COVID."

Steven Magee

Summary

So what have I learned since I have been researching supplements? The human body accumulates damage as it ages from environmental exposures, injuries and infections. Altitude sickness and coronavirus infections are very similar and can cause comparable damage throughout the body from hypoxia. It can make a person sensitized to just a small change in altitude or air pressure. Nutritional supplements can offset some of this damage by correcting malnutrition issues in the body and detoxifying toxins the damaged body is producing.

It is no secret the medical profession struggles with long COVID patients. They appear to stay sickly under their care and throwing prescription drugs and medical devices at their unusual health conditions can make them sicker! Many of my long COVID symptoms were misdiagnosed during years of visits to numerous doctors. I was never referred to a nutritionist, despite having serious food intolerance for years.

The mental health profession were very disappointing. I was surprised at how bad they were! They will diagnose you with a range of mental health conditions and start prescribing you potent brain drugs. When you tell them the brain drugs are making you sicker, they tell you to take more! The treatment was so bad from them that I had to stop using them to protect my own health and safety!

Mental illness is a common diagnosis that doctors fall back onto when they do not understand what is wrong with the patient. You need to be very careful about interacting with doctors with this diagnosis. If you start talking about poisoning with them, they may say it is your mental illness making you paranoid and you may get locked up in the mental health hospital! Be very careful about your interactions with doctors once you have a mental illness diagnosis! They have the power to institutionalize you.

I was attending an army of doctors from 2015 to 2021 with long COVID symptoms. Many were at the university research hospital. They could not accurately diagnose me. What was I telling them? The sickness I have feels like altitude sickness! I have looked up my symptoms and it matches poisoning! They could not diagnose altitude hypersensitivity and ammonia poisoning. Nothing showed up on their many medical tests to indicate these conditions were present. This is how my treatment went:

- Lung damage and asthma was treated with numerous inhalers. The actual treatment was to move to a rural sea level area.

- Sleep apnea and bruxism were treated with an anti-back device, stimulants, CPAP and BiPAP machines. The CPAP and BiPAP machines had been given to me with the pressure setting too high and were actually making me sicker! The actual treatment was to move to sea level, sleep on my front and take magnesium.

- Mental illness was treated with potent brain drugs. The actual treatment was to identify the altitude hypersensitivity and ammonia poisoning, take amino acids and move to sea level.

- Fatigue was treated with stimulants. The actual treatment was to identify nutritional deficiencies, food intolerance and disrupted circadian rhythms, and take amino acids, move to sea level and live in a tent outside for several months.

- Heart arrhythmia was being treated with numerous prescription medications. The actual treatment was nutritional support for the heart and move to sea level.

- Gastrointestinal problems were treated with a colonoscopy and removal of a polyp. They got part of the treatment right. The full treatment was live culture support from yogurt, nutritional support, daily exercise, a cooler environment and move to sea level.

- Fungal toenails were treated by removing the toenails and painting an anti-fungal onto the new nails which did not work. The correct treatment appears to be an oral anti-fungal for several months, painting an anti-fungal onto the toenails, treating the ammonia poisoning and move to sea level.

- Food intolerance was never treated. The correct treatment was to adopt a comprehensive nutritional support system that included amino acids, a low protein diet and move to sea level.

- Altitude sickness was never treated. The correct treatment was to move to sea level and take L-Carnitine and glycine.

- Poisoning was never treated. The correct treatment was arginine, citrulline and lysine nutritional supplementation, detoxify from heavy metals poisoning and move to sea level.

My treatment from the doctors ranged from almost nothing through to lots of prescription drugs. The treatment varied between each doctor. Some were watching how my health was degrading and monitoring it, while others were trying to use prescription drugs to fix it. I had one doctor that was trying to tell me it was "All in my mind!". I left that doctor after hearing that.

Be aware the modern medical profession has no real incentive to fix you. Financially, the doctor is in a much better position if you stay sick, because you will be a regular at the office and will be producing a nice income for the doctor!

There are no doubts that the modern medical system is under the influence of pharmaceutical companies. Many of their expensive drugs work no better than nutritional supplements! But the prescriptions may come with nasty side effects. Some of my prescription medications were $500 per month for each medicine!

By the time I was done with the medical profession in 2021, I had been under the care of numerous primary care doctors, numerous specialist doctors and I had been attending the four main hospitals in Tucson including the university research hospital.

At the age of fifty-three I will never be cured of permanent biological damage. I was fortunate I had some lucky breaks that improved my mental functioning to the point I could correctly self diagnose my symptoms. One of these was my ex-girlfriend switching out my diet to a gluten free one. Had this not happened, I would still be misdiagnosed!

I call my disease "Magee's Disease", as I have not been able to find a medical condition in the published medical literature that covers the full range of health issues I had. As such, I believe Magee's disease is a new and previously undocumented health condition in the general population. This explains why all of the numerous doctors I saw were unable to make a diagnosis of Magee's disease and prescribe the correct treatment.

My recovery has been so successful that I have not been to a doctors office since I left Arizona in July 2021. I have medical insurance in Hawaii and I have never needed to use it in almost two years. I do not have a primary care doctor. At the peak of the sickness in Tucson, I was averaging a doctors visit every few weeks! I was under the care of a wide range of specialist doctors at the time.

My other books provide further information on health and you may want to consider reading them:

- COVID Supplements.

- Pandemic Supplements.

- Magee's Disease.

- Curing Electromagnetic Hypersensitivity.

- Toxic Altitude.

- Toxic Electricity.

- Toxic Health.

- Toxic Light.

- Solar Radiation, Global Warming, and Human Disease.

I hope you enjoyed this book and I wish you the very best of health.

"I was surprised the USA medical profession could not diagnose low blood oxygen levels, sensitivity to abnormal air, food intolerance, malnutrition, a urea cycle disorder, altitude hypersensitivity, loss of circadian rhythm and loss of moonlight synchronization."

Steven Magee

References

Books:

- Brain Longevity by Dharma Singh Khalsa.

- Brain Maker: The Power of Gut Microbes to Heal and Protect Your Brain - for Life by David Perlmutter with Kristin Loberg.

- HEAVY METALS DETOX: The fast-track to a healthier version of YOU! by James Lilley.

- No Grain, No Pain: A 30-Day Diet for Eliminating the Root Cause of Chronic Pain by Peter Osborne.

- Prescription For Nutritional Healing by James F. Balch, MD & Phyllis A Balch, CNC.

- The Complete Low-FODMAP Diet: A Revolutionary Plan for Managing IBS and Other Digestive Disorders by Sue Shepherd.

- The Pill Book Guide to Natural Medicines by Michael Murray N.D.

- The Plant Paradox - The Hidden Dangers in "Healthy" Foods That Cause Disease and Weight Gain by Dr. Steven R Gundry MD.

- Understanding Nutrition by Ellie Whitney & Sharon Rady Rolfes.

- Wheat Belly by William Davis.

Internet:

- Dietary supplement:
  - https://en.wikipedia.org/wiki/Dietary_supplement

- Linus Pauling Institute's Micronutrient Information Center:
  - https://lpi.oregonstate.edu/mic/
- NIH Dietary Supplement Fact Sheets:
  - https://ods.od.nih.gov/factsheets/list-all/
- Mayo Clinic nutrition and healthy eating:
  - https://www.mayoclinic.org/healthy-lifestyle/nutrition-and-healthy-eating/basics/nutrition-basics/hlv-20049477
- The Nutrition Source at Harvard College:
  - https://www.hsph.harvard.edu/nutritionsource/
- WebMD Vitamins & Supplements:
  - https://www.webmd.com/vitamins/index

"I found my correct diagnosis in books and on the internet."

Steven Magee

Most At Risk Of Hypoxia

The most at risk of hypoxia illnesses and diseases are:

- Space.
  - Astronauts.
  - Tourists.
- Aviation workers.
  - Pilots.
  - Airline cabin crew.
  - Frequent fliers.
- High altitude astronomy workers.
- Winter sports.
  - Skiers.
  - Snowboarders.
- Mountain hikers.
- High altitude hikers.
- Mountain workers.
  - Lodges.
  - Resorts.
  - Some national parks.
- Forest workers.
- People that live in altitude cities.
- Drivers and truckers.
- Radio and television transmitter workers.
- Cell phone tower workers.

- People with pre-existing health conditions.

- People with sea level adapted genetics.

- People with a hole in the heart (ASD).

- People that have breathed industrial gasses.

- People that have breathed medical gasses.

- People that live inside poorly ventilated homes with gas appliances.

- People that have been exposed to hypoxic environments.

- People that have had a coronavirus infection.

- People with Long COVID.

"Truckers that drive all over the USA are often in hypoxic environments!"

Steven Magee

Acknowledgments

This book was influenced by:

- Those that are developing the important science of environmental health and bringing it to the masses.

- My family for providing support during my prolonged and mysterious illness.

"Mysterious disabling illnesses will make you dependent on people."

Steven Magee

About The Author

About Steven Magee CEng MIET BEng Hons, member of Environmental Radiation LLC:

Steven was born in the United Kingdom (UK) and started his career at one of the largest university research and teaching hospitals in Europe. Working in the electrical engineering group, he obtained a Bachelors with Honors in Electrical and Electronic Engineering. Human health was a strong draw and he moved into the biomedical team, serving the regions hospitals. During this time he developed a fascination for human illness and disease and the causes of it, many of which were not understood.

He joined the Isaac Newton Group of Telescopes in 1999 and went to live in La Palma. La Palma is part of the Canary Islands, governed by Spain. During this time he worked with the leading European astronomers and developed his astronomical and optics skills. He became fluent in Spanish and their culture.

In 2001 he became a Chartered Electrical Engineer and joined the W. M. Keck Observatory in Hawaii. This was the world's leading astronomical facility and home to the world's two largest segmented mirror telescopes. Steven developed segmented optics and interferometry skills while working alongside world leading astronomers. He was the assistant to Nobel Prize winners including the fourth woman to win the prize in physics, Andrea Ghez. During this time Steven constructed his own off-grid solar powered home in the last of the traditional Hawaiian fishing villages in Miloli'i, Hawaii. He learned Hawaiian Pidgin English and the Hawaiian culture during his time there.

In 2006, Steven became the Director of the MDM Observatory in Sells, Arizona, USA. Working for Columbia University and later, Dartmouth College, he developed the facility to modern standards. He learned an appreciation of the Native Americans and their culture from the Tohono O'odham Nation.

In 2008, Steven joined the solar power revolution that was sweeping the USA and commissioned the largest CIGS thin film solar photovoltaic installation in the world.

A year later he became the Florida Power and Light (FPL) Manager of the DeSoto Next Generation Solar Energy Center, which was the largest solar photovoltaic utility power generation plant ever built in the USA. The system rated power was quoted as 25,000,000 watts AC with over 90,500 solar modules that were mounted to 158 single-axis tracker systems in three hundred acres of land and it was opened by President Obama.

He went on to develop the solar photovoltaic team for a large international company.

In 2010 he started to research radiation and publish the leading books on the subject.

He became a USA citizen in 2017 and continues to be interested in global radiation health effects and how it impacts over seven billion people on planet Earth.

"I had a very interesting career that sent me into ill health and onto disability."

Steven Magee

Author Contact

This is the Environmental Radiation LLC website:

- www.environmentalradiation.com

You can follow the Twitter feed at:

- Steven Magee @EnvironmentEMR
- https://twitter.com/EnvironmentEMR

The Facebook page is:

- https://www.facebook.com/EnvironmentEMR

You may find my other books useful:

Altitude Sickness

- **Magee's Disease:** Magee's Disease, Summit Brain, Altitude Sickness, COVID-19 and Long COVID are all related. This book delves into the silent world of hypoxia and what it can do to people. The failings of the modern medical profession are examined and solutions to the hypoxic Magee's Disease are explored.

- **Summit Brain:** Summit Brain is a term used to describe the health issues that appear in people that commute to very high altitude. This book explores the biological reasons that cause Summit Brain to occur. Recovery from Summit Brain can be achieved and solutions are explored for underlying conditions that doctors may have missed.

Architecture

- **Solar Reflections for Architects, Engineers, and Human Health**: This book is a comprehensive collection of images, diagrams, and notes that document the effects of sunlight in architecture. This is essential information for architects, engineers, and the medical profession. The discovery of the "Multiple-Sun" effect in architecture is detailed and this book is illustrated in color.

Circadian Rhythms & Sleep Disorders

- **Night Shift Recovery:** Unusual work shifts may lead to the development of Shift Work Disorder. Shift work is well known for its ability to degrade human health. Recovery can be achieved and solutions are explored for underlying conditions that doctors may have missed.

Climate Change

- **Solar Radiation, Global Warming, and Human Disease**: This book examines the modern development of the Earth and the potential impacts on global warming and human disease. The destruction of the forests for modern agricultural use appears to have effects that are not fully understood and these are explored. Radiation deficiency and radiation overloading are investigated to see if they are factors in many illnesses and diseases.

Human Health

- **Hypoxia, Mental Illness & Chronic Fatigue**: This book examines the many aspects of hypoxia that may lead to the development of mental illness and chronic fatigue. Modern society is filled with hypoxia experiences that are well known for their ability to affect brain functioning and energy levels. Solutions are explored for underlying conditions that doctors may have missed.

- **Solar Radiation – A Cause of Illness and Cancer?** Illness and cancers have become part of our modern culture. It has been discovered that extremely high levels of man-made solar radiation exist in modern society. Could this be the one of the causes of illness and cancers? This book examines the increase in solar radiation and applies it to human health.

Nutrition

- **COVID Supplements:** Steven Magee became disabled by a mystery flu-like sickness he caught from an international university professor. During the COVID-19 pandemic, he realized his mysterious range of symptoms matched a new sickness called Long COVID. This book explores the science behind the nutritional supplements he used to recover his mental and physical health.

- **Long COVID Supplements:** Steven Magee became disabled by a mystery flu-like sickness he caught from an international university professor. During the COVID-19 pandemic, he realized his mysterious range of symptoms matched a new sickness called Long COVID. This book explores the Long COVID science behind the nutritional supplements he used to recover his mental and physical health.

- **Pandemic Supplements:** Steven Magee became disabled by a mystery flu-like sickness he caught from an international university professor. During the COVID-19 pandemic, he realized his mysterious range of symptoms matched a new sickness called Long COVID. This book explores the nutritional supplements he used to recover his mental and physical health.

Toxicity

- **Toxic Altitude:** Toxic Altitude explores the biological reasons that cause Altitude Sickness to occur in sea level adapted humans. Recovery from the long term effects of Altitude Sickness can be achieved and solutions are explored for underlying conditions that doctors may have missed.

- **Toxic Electricity:** Random aches and pains? Fatigue? Insomnia? Facial pains? Irregular heartbeats? Sick kids? Relationship problems? Blotchy skin? Anxiety? Toxic electricity takes a look at the electrical system and asks the question: Is this one of the most toxic endeavors that humanity has ever engaged in?

- **Toxic Health:** Toxic Health takes a look at the pollution that may be in your local environment and relates it to the health problems that it can cause. Pollution in the human environment is only just starting to be understood and something as innocent as light may be able to make you really ill! There are many examples of commonplace items in your environment that may have the ability to affect your health. In particular, we will investigate if modern city life is the most toxic thing of all to the modern human!

- **Toxic Light:** Toxic Light takes a look at the light pollution that may be in your local environment and relates it to the health problems that it may cause. Light in the human environment is only just starting to be understood and something as innocent as your sunglasses may be able to make you ill! There are many examples of commonplace items in your environment that may have the ability to affect your health. Get ready for enlightenment about the most important human nutrient of light!

Forensics

- **Electrical Forensics:** Electrical Forensics examines the many aspects of electricity, electronics and wireless communications that may lead to unusual behaviors to occur in humans. Electromagnetic interference is well known for its ability to affect mental functioning and human health. Electrical Forensics demonstrates how to identify toxic electromagnetic environments that may be the root cause of accidents and crimes.

- **Health Forensics:** Health Forensics examines the many aspects of modern society that may lead to unusual behaviors to occur in humans. Modern society has adopted habits that are well known for their ability to affect mental functioning and human health. Health Forensics demonstrates how to identify toxic human environments that may be the root cause of accidents and crimes.

- **Light Forensics**: Light Forensics examines the many aspects of modern lighting that may lead to unusual behaviors to occur in humans. Modern society has adopted optical products that are well known for their ability to affect mental functioning and human health. Light Forensics demonstrates how to identify toxic light that may be the root cause of accidents and crimes.

Religion

- **Solar Radiation, the Book of Revelations, and the Era of Light – Part 1:** Welcome to the Era of Light! Light has long been known to be essential nourishment for the human body. We will explore the different types of light that are present on Earth and relate it to human health and nature. Light is discussed extensively in the Bible and we will see if we can associate our findings to it. Finally, we will investigate if the Industrial Revolution has created the ultimate toxin of poisonous sunlight!

Professional

- **Engineering Science and Education Journal Volume: 11, Issue: 4, Active Control Systems for Large Segmented Optical Mirrors:** A new generation of optical telescopes is on the drawing board. These will be true giants with primary mirrors having a diameter of up to 100 meters. The technology that will enable this revolution to take place was developed at the W. M. Keck Observatory in Hawaii, where the world's largest segmented mirrors are in daily use. This article looks at how the W. M. Keck Observatory proved the mirror technology that will be behind this new generation of telescopes.

Solar Photovoltaic

- **Complete Solar Photovoltaics for Residential, Commercial, and Utility Systems:** Steven Magee has combined his three top selling books on solar power systems into one edition. Complete Solar Photovoltaics will train you on solar photovoltaics and show you how to design grid connected solar photovoltaic power systems. Operations and maintenance is detailed to enable you to have a complete understanding of solar photovoltaics from start to finish.

- **Solar Photovoltaics for Consumers, Utilities, and Investors:** This book details solar photovoltaic systems for consumers, utilities and investors. This would encompass residential, commercial and utility systems that are connected to the utility grid. There is a discussion of the different technologies available for the consumer and their advantages and disadvantages. For the utilities, there is invaluable advice on planning and constructing large projects. For the investor, forward looking statements try to predict the future of solar photovoltaics.

- **Solar Photovoltaic Training for Residential, Commercial, and Utility Systems:** This book details solar photovoltaic training for those who are interested in this area and also for those who are already working in the field. This would encompass residential, commercial, and utility systems that are connected to the utility grid. It is a comprehensive overview of a rapidly growing world of solar photovoltaic power generation technology.

- **Solar Photovoltaic Design for Residential, Commercial, and Utility Systems:** This book details how to design reliable solar photovoltaic power generation systems from a residential system, progressing to a commercial system, and finishing at the largest utility power generation systems. By following the guidelines in this book and your local solar photovoltaic electrical codes, you will be able to design trouble free solar power systems that give many years of reliable operation. When designed well, solar photovoltaic power generation is an excellent source of electrical power that results in much lower electricity bills, the power company will even refund you for the excess energy generated by your system if it is large enough. Building a grid tied solar power system is a relatively easy task. Given the large amount of government and electrical utility financial incentives that are available, it is a great time to join in the solar power revolution that is taking place in the world today.

- **Solar Photovoltaic Operation and Maintenance for Residential, Commercial, and Utility Systems:** This book details how to operate and maintain residential, commercial, and utility solar photovoltaic systems that are connected to the utility grid. By following the guidelines in this book you will be able to operate and maintain solar power systems that should give many years of reliable operation. Invaluable trouble shooting advice will aid in returning your system to full operation in the event of a problem.

- **Solar Photovoltaic DC Calculations for Residential, Commercial, and Utility Systems:** This book details how to run calculations for the DC circuit of solar photovoltaic systems. This would encompass residential, commercial, and utility systems that are connected to the utility grid. It covers the range of conditions that solar photovoltaic modules are exposed to throughout the year and shows how to incorporate these into an effective DC circuit that is well designed and reliable.

- **Solar Photovoltaic Resource for Residential, Commercial, and Utility Systems:** This book is a resource of information that is used in the solar photovoltaic field. This would encompass residential, commercial, and utility systems that are connected to the utility grid. It is a comprehensive collection of notes, diagrams, pictures and charts for a rapidly growing world of solar photovoltaic power generation technology. This book is illustrated in color.

Solar Radiation

- **Solar Irradiance and Insolation for Power Systems:** This book is a resource of information that is used in the solar power generation field. This would encompass residential, commercial, and utility systems that are connected to the utility grid. It is a comprehensive collection of notes, diagrams, pictures, and charts for a rapidly growing world of solar photovoltaic power generation technology. This book is illustrated in color.

- **Solar Site Selection for Power Systems:** This book is a comprehensive collection of images, diagrams, and notes that document the effects of light and heat in the solar power generation field. This would encompass residential, commercial, and utility systems that are connected to the utility grid. This is essential information for a rapidly growing world of solar power generation technology. This book is illustrated in color.

You can search "Steven Magee Books" for the very latest publications.

www.youtube.com videos supporting the ideas in the books can be found by searching StevenMageeBooks:

- https://www.youtube.com/user/StevenMageeBooks

"Writing books is by far the most interesting thing I have done in life."

Steven Magee

Book Reviews

Complete Solar Photovoltaics for Residential, Commercial, and Utility Systems rated 5 out of 5 stars.

Reviewed by Amanda Bassett on December 4, 2015 titled "Perfect read".

Perfect for solar farm studies. Takes the reader from basics who doesn't know a sausage about electricity to turning it into a business. We are considering doing just this in Arizona ourselves.

Curing Electromagnetic Hypersensitivity rated 5 out of 5 stars.

Reviewed by Ann on on January 31, 2015 titled "Don't miss the message here folks!".

This book says a lot abut the importance of not only avoiding radiation but the necessity of taking steps to replenish and rebalance the body's own electrical system in order to build resistance to the unavoidable radiation exposures that we live with in this world. I have suffered with EHS and MCS and over the years I have gotten the most improvement by tracking my nutrient/mineral levels and supplementing accordingly. I am not surprised that the author has gotten his health back by "charging his battery, " so to speak. I have always believed that the most effective way to prevent or cure disease is to improve the "terrain" of the body. Thanks to the author for pointing this out and sharing the specifics!

Electrical Forensics rated 5 out of 5 stars.

Review by John Puccetti on October 27, 2013 titled "Dangers of electricity"

Steven has made many of the health problems of our century known in his book. But what will we do is this information? We live in a corporate dictatorship that masquerades as democracy.

Health Forensics rated 5 out of 5 stars.

Reviewed by honesT on July 26, 2014 titled "Incredible insights you would have never thought of :O".

Incredible insights, seriously Steve nails it again. If your just an average person looking for some insight about the whole EMF thing this is for you 100%. If your a seasoned EMF pro looking for some new insights this book is worth it`s weight in gold and you will, I have no doubt in my mind take in new knowledge that will no doubt open doors. You do not have to read this book from cover to cover, just pick any chapter read and be amazed what you learn. So many areas are covered in this book, it`s really like a mini encyclopedia for EMF and how that`s affecting our surroundings that in turn affect our body, mind and emotions. I really can`t say enough I mean just look at the price it`s practically free :]

Solar Photovoltaic Training for Residential, Commercial and Utility Systems rated 5 out of 5 stars.

Reviewed by Kyle William Loshure on November 13, 2016 titled "Solar power is #1"

Thank you for your work!

Solar Radiation, Global Warming and Human Disease rated 5 out of 5 stars.

Reviewed by Donato Cobarrubias on October 4, 2014 titled "Five Stars"

Great book and great info! I learned a lot!

Toxic Electricity rated 5 out of 5 stars.

Review by Sam Wieder on December 13, 2013 titled "A Most Illuminating, Educational, and Helpful Book"

Toxic Electricity provides a clear and comprehensive description of the many ways in which electrical fields impact human health and offers simple steps that anyone can take to live a more vibrant life in our electrically toxic world. The author does a masterful job of presenting some fairly complex concepts in a way that is easily understandable. Reading this book will give you a deeper understanding of how unseen radiation in your living and working environment may be impacting you. If you've been battling different health challenges or are chronically tired for no apparent reason, this book may very well open your eyes to some answers that will help you regain your health and your life.

Toxic Light rated 5 out of 5 stars.

Titled "Five Stars".

Reviewed by Amazon Customer on September 17, 2018

Great book, lots of information about light you never hear about anywhere.

"When I saw the five star reviews appearing, I knew the research was progressing in the right direction."

Steven Magee